Asperger Syndrome
• An Owner's Manual 2 •

Asperger Syndrome
• An Owner's Manual 2 •
For Older Adolescents and Adults

What You, Your Parents and Friends, and
Your Employer, Need to Know

Ellen S. Heller Korin, M.Ed.

APC

Autism Asperger Publishing Co.
P.O. Box 23173
Shawnee Mission, Kansas 66283-0173
www.asperger.net

©2007 Autism Asperger Publishing Company
P.O. Box 23173
Shawnee Mission, KS 66283-0173
www.asperger.net

Publisher's Cataloging-in-Publication

Korin, Ellen S. Heller.

Asperger syndrome--an owner's manual for older adolescents and adults : what you, your parents and friends, and your employer, need to know / Ellen S. Heller Korin. -- 1st ed. -- Shawnee Mission, Kan. : Autism Asperger Pub. Co., 2007.

p. ; cm.

ISBN: 978-1-934575-06-2
LCCN: 2007932563

Includes bibliographical references.
"An interactive guide and workbook."
Audience: adolescents/young adults and their parents and teachers.
"In the spring of 2006 [the author] published 'Asperger Syndrome, an owner's manual : what you, your parents and your teachers need to know'. ...This then is volume 2: What you, your family and friends, and your employer, need to know."--Intro.

   1. Asperger's syndrome in adolescence. 2. Asperger's syndrome in adolescence--Handbooks, manuals, etc. 3. Autistic children--Behavior modification. 4. Asperger's syndrome in adolescence--Treatment. I. Title. II. Asperger syndrome, an owner's manual : what you, your parents and your teachers need to know.

RJ506.A9 .K672 2007
618.92/858832--dc22   0708

Designed in Helvetica Neue and American Typewriter.

Printed in the United States of America.

"I am only one, but still I am one.

I cannot do everything, but still I can do something; and because I cannot do everything, I will not refuse to do something that I can do."

– Helen Keller

DEDICATION

For Sarah, in memory of her Panta,

My brother, David,

And for his namesake ... Danielle Emily.

For Jonathan – the wind beneath my wings ...

For Alexandra – who lights up the world around her

And in memory of my parents, Ruth Klemas Heller Kalle and Alexander Heller.

ACKNOWLEDGMENTS

Once again I thank all of the wonderful people in the AS community with whom I have had the privilege of working. My life has been enriched immeasurably by our work together. I delight in your triumphs. I also want to thank Kirsten McBride and all the folks at AAPC, my staunch supporters at AANE and, most of all, my friends and family, especially my devoted husband, Jonathan, and the light of my life, Alexandra.

Table of Contents

Introduction 1
   Overview of the Book 1
   Getting Ready to Use the Workbook 3
   People I Can Trust to Help Me 4
   A Word About Parents 4

Part 1: Understanding Asperger Syndrome 5
  The Spectrum: Definitions of Autism and Asperger Syndrome 6
   Asperger Syndrome Defined – What Is It? 7
   What Does All This Mean? 8
   One and Only One 9
   Common Characteristics 9
  Understanding Your Profile 11
   Typical Goals/Atypical Mind 11
   What's Your Independent Life Skills Timetable? 12
  Your Vision and Goals: Vision – Goal – Plan (VGP) 15
   Create a Vision 15
   Identify Your Goals 20
  Assessment 25
   How Prepared Are You to Pursue Your Goals? 25
   Independent Life Skills Assessment 29
   Self-Appraisal 34

Part 2: Putting It All Together 39
  From Profile to Plan 40
  Coaching 42
   Why Coaching? 42
   Coaching in a Nutshell 43
  Getting Started 44
   Set Priorities 44
   Create a Plan 46
  Developing Needed Skills 50
   Strategies 50
   PAPI Model 51
   More Skills to Develop/More Strategies to Learn 59
   Applying Skills You Have Learned: Combining Vision-Goal-Plan (VGP) with PAPI....71
  On the Road to Success 87
   Roadblocks to Change 87
   Evading Roadblocks 87
   Your Core Identity 88
   More Roadblocks 89
   Another Note About Parents 91

Disclosure: To Do or Not to Do 92
Final Thoughts 98
Appendix 99

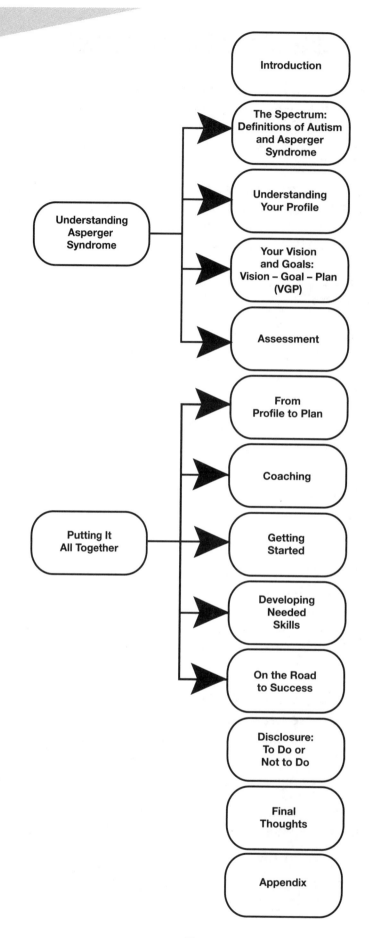

INTRODUCTION

In the spring of 2006 I published *Asperger Syndrome, An Owner's Manual: What You, Your Parents and Your Teachers Need to Know*. As I worked on this resource primarily for middle-school age children with AS, I knew that I would want to create something for the older adolescents and adults with whom I work. This, then, is Volume 2: *What You, Your Family and Friends, and Your Employer, Need to Know*. Like its predecessor, it is an interactive workbook designed to assist users in identifying their unique profiles in order to devise appropriate and customized interventions and strategies. It can be completed independently, but in most cases is better done with the assistance of a coach, therapist, or advocate. Parents are also likely to be important contributors, even for adults.

The book is based on the premise that, despite a common diagnosis, each individual with Asperger Syndrome (AS) is genuinely unique and that to create successful plans for living, learning and, yes, loving, with AS, strategies must be derived from the individual's profile. Generic strategies don't always apply; one size does not fit all.

This volume is intended for older adolescents (16+) and for adults on the spectrum who have the desire to enhance their quality of life and achieve unmet goals. It is most appropriate for people on the "upper" end of the spectrum (Asperger Syndrome and high-functioning autism). It will require users to

- Work on identifying behaviors they exhibit that may be hindering them;
- Identify neurotypical behavior;
- Try out the "un-natural" in order to improve in certain areas.

Self-awareness, like so many other skills, can be acquired through hard work and practice. Motivation and willingness to try are the key requisites for success with this workbook. What I hope users will accomplish is an understanding of the ways in which Asperger Syndrome affects them personally and to use that information to make plans, adjustments and strategies that will lead them to accomplish self-set goals and improve their life situations.

Overview of the Book

This workbook is divided into two main parts. The focus of the first section is on assisting users in gathering information, both general and specific, about Asperger Syndrome and about themselves. The second part of the book guides users in a process of translating the information they have gathered into plans for achieving the goals they have identified. Within this section you will find strategies, suggestions and adjustments that can be helpful for minimizing constraints and maximizing opportunities to achieve goals. When knowledge and understanding connect with goals and strategic planning, you can anticipate more control of life circumstances, ideally, resulting in a more fulfilling life experience.

We will use the nonagram to visually guide us through the workbook. The nonagram, or nine-pointed star, is a symbol of achievement and completeness. As the last single digit in the decimal number system, nine is a number of fulfillment, fullness and limits. As we proceed through the book, we will complete more and more of the star, which will be represented by grey shading.

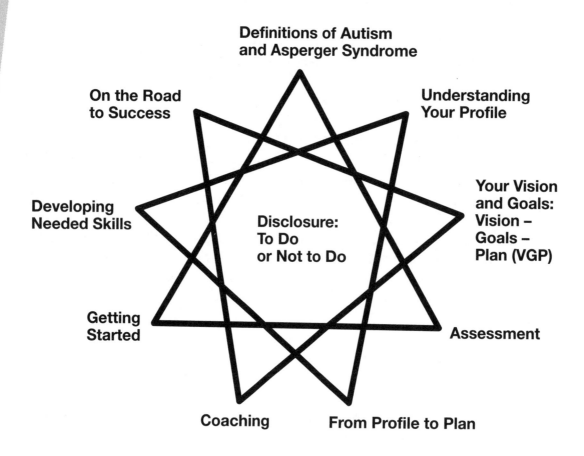

Definitions of Autism and Asperger Syndrome

On the Road to Success

Understanding Your Profile

Developing Needed Skills

Disclosure: To Do or Not to Do

Your Vision and Goals: Vision – Goals – Plan (VGP)

Getting Started

Assessment

Coaching

From Profile to Plan

=

More Control/Higher Quality of Life

Getting Ready to Use the Workbook

What you will need:

- an open mind
- a pencil or erasable pen
- a small notebook or
- a set of index cards (different colors) and a metal ring to hang the cards on, or a pocket coupon organizer
- a friend or relative you trust to help you and corroborate your ideas

In the course of utilizing this workbook, you are likely to generate lots of information and potential aids or strategies. Some of this information will be recorded right in the workbook. However, you may want to devise a "storage" system of "cue" (index) cards or a strategy notebook for recording and later more easily accessing your interventions and plans. If you use index cards, file them in a pocket coupon organizer that you have customized (substitute categories such as "greetings," "self-care," "interviews," etc., for "meats," "cereals"), or get a metal ring on which you can hang the cards once you have punched a hole in each. If you choose a notebook, try to find one that will be easily transportable and is durable. A small loose-leaf notebook works well.

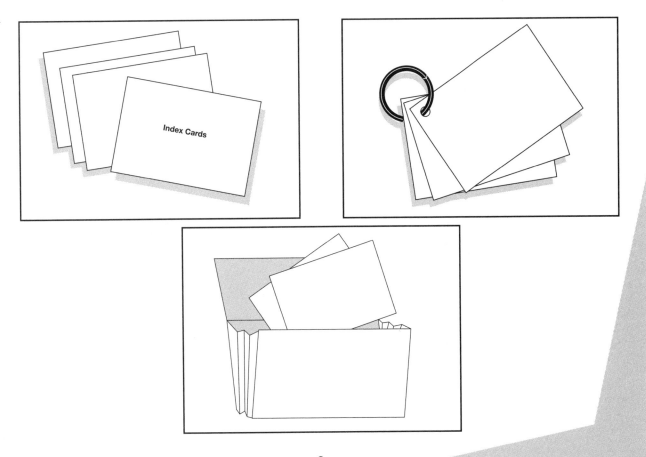

People I Can Trust to Help Me

Many of the tasks you are completing in this workbook may be challenging for you, especially at first. Therefore, you may find it helpful to identify one or two "allies" who can help you. Be sure that the people you ask to help will be honest, yet sensitive to your feelings. You must feel confident that they will not share your personal information with others, unless you give them permission and it is otherwise appropriate. They should know you well and want to help. You can use their help to generate ideas and information or to corroborate what you have generated. People who might be potential allies could be a close relative, a helping person such as a counselor, a family friend or a friend of long standing.

A Word About Parents

If you live with your parents (or if they are still an active part of your life), it is essential to obtain their understanding and support as you try making some of the changes discussed here. What *support* means varies dramatically from situation to situation. While one person with AS may need protection, another may need more of a "tough love" approach. But in all cases, it is important that parents

- share the goal of independence for their adult child,

- learn to tolerate the pace of their child's development, and

- accept that their child may not follow the conventional path at the conventional pace.

PART 1: UNDERSTANDING ASPERGER SYNDROME

The Spectrum: Definitions of Autism and Asperger Syndrome

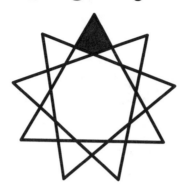

According to the DSM-IV (*Diagnostic and Statistical Manual of Mental Disorders, 4th Edition* – a commonly used diagnostic manual published by the American Psychiatric Association), autism (autism spectrum disorders, referred to as ASD) is classified as a pervasive developmental disorder and is defined as follows:

A. A total of six (or more) items from (1), (2), and (3), with at least two from (1), and one each from (2) and (3).

1. Qualitative impairment in social interaction, as manifested by at least two of the following:

    a. marked impairment in the use of multiple nonverbal behaviors such as eye-to-eye gaze, facial expression, body postures, and gestures, to regulate social interaction.
    b. failure to develop peer relationships appropriate to developmental level.
    c. a lack of spontaneous seeking to share enjoyment, interests or achievements with other people, for example, by a lack of showing, bringing or pointing out objects of interest.
    d. lack of social or emotional reciprocity.

2. Qualitative impairments in communication as manifested by at least one of the following:

    a. delay in, or total lack of, the development of spoken language not accompanied by an attempt to compensate through alternative modes of communication such as gesture or mime
    b. in individuals with adequate speech, marked impairment in the ability to initiate or sustain a conversation with others
    c. lack of varied, spontaneous, make-believe play or social imitative play appropriate to developmental level

3. Restricted, repetitive and stereotyped patterns of behavior, interests and activities, as manifested by at least one of the following:

a. encompassing preoccupation with one or more stereotyped and restricted patterns of interest that is abnormal either in intensity or focus

b. apparently inflexible adherence to specific nonfunctional routines or rituals

c. stereotyped and repetitive motor mannerisms, for example, hand or finger flapping or twisting, or complex whole-body movements

d. persistent preoccupation with parts of objects

B. Delays or abnormal functioning in at least one of the following areas, with onset prior to age 3 years:

1. social interaction
2. language as used in social communication
3. symbolic or imaginative play

C. The disturbance is not better accounted for by Rett's Disorder or Childhood Disintegrative Disorder

Autism as defined by the DSM is now thought to be one end of a spectrum or range of disorders, with classic autism the most severe form and Asperger Syndrome and nonverbal learning disabilities thought to be less severe forms.

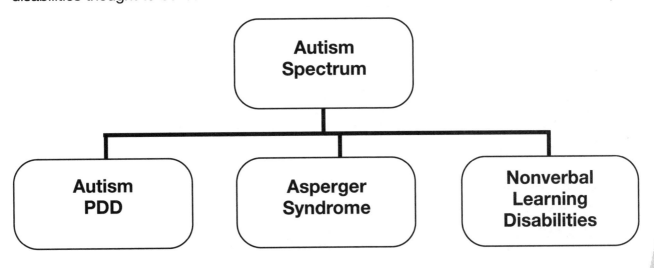

Asperger Syndrome Defined – What Is It?

Within the broad category of pervasive developmental disorder also lies Asperger Syndrome, defined in the DSM-IV as:

A. Qualitative impairment in social interaction, as manifested by at least two of the following:

1. marked impairments in the use of multiple nonverbal behaviors such as eye-to-eye gaze, facial expression, body postures, and gestures to regulate social interaction

2. failure to develop peer relationships appropriate to developmental level
3. a lack of spontaneous seeking to share enjoyment, interests, or achievements with other people (e.g., by a lack of showing, bringing, or pointing out objects of interest to other people)
4. lack of social or emotional reciprocity

B. Restricted repetitive and stereotyped patterns of behavior, interests, and activities, as manifested by at least one of the following:

1. encompassing preoccupation with one or more stereotyped and restricted patterns of interest that is abnormal either in intensity or focus
2. apparently inflexible adherence to specific, nonfunctional routines or rituals
3. stereotyped and repetitive motor mannerisms (e.g., hand or finger flapping or twisting, or complex whole-body movements)
4. persistent preoccupation with parts of objects

C. The disturbance causes clinically significant impairment in social, occupational, or other important areas of functioning

D. There is no clinically significant general delay in language (e.g., single words used by age 2 years, communicative phrases used by age 3 years)

E. There is no clinically significant delay in cognitive development or in the development of age-appropriate self-help skills, adaptive behavior (other than social interaction), and curiosity about the environment in childhood

F. Criteria are not met for another specific Pervasive Developmental Disorder or Schizophrenia

It is important to note that many people exhibit some, but not all, of the characteristics needed to qualify for the diagnosis of autism, or an uneven distribution of characteristics. When this occurs, the diagnosis of pervasive developmental disorder-not otherwise specified (PDD-NOS) is applied. PDD-NOS is considered a "sub-threshold" or an atypical form of autism.

What Does All This Mean?

In lay terms, what this says is that to officially "qualify" for the diagnosis of Asperger Syndrome, one must exhibit deficits (at least two) in the area of social interaction (see A above) and must also exhibit perseverative (including special interests) behaviors, such as those listed under B above. The symptoms must be sufficient to cause substantial interference in one or more areas of life functioning. However, there must be an absence of significant language and cognitive delays in the developmental history of the AS "candidate."

One and Only One

In reality, each person with AS is truly unique. Although there are some "common characteristics," the combination of these characteristics and the expression thereof are totally individual. While it is sometimes helpful to obtain an "official" diagnosis, the diagnosis itself does not give sufficient information (specificity) about the ways in which AS affects the individual: what "symptoms" s/he exhibits; what may have been factors historically but are no longer as significant, etc.

People with AS or "near AS" are unique individuals with a wide spectrum of behaviors and abilities as well as constraints in certain areas. The degree to which AS impacts and/or limits them covers a broad range and is subject to change. Thus, the DSM-IV definition given above may be viewed as a starting point, a framework as it were, but it is not a true description of the person with AS. As one young adult put it, "the diagnosis is a road map"; it leads you in the direction of information and resources.

A psychiatrist is generally consulted in order to determine if a diagnosis of an ASD is appropriate. To find a psychiatrist who has experience with ASD, you might consult with people at a local ASD organization. These folks tend to be wonderful sources of information and support.

To find local resources, check out http://www.udel.edu/bkirby/asperger/localsupport.htm This is a terrific website overall, and this particular page lists resources by state.

Despite the variability in profiles, there are some common characteristics that are associated with Asperger Syndrome, as outlined below.

Common Characteristics

Even though not seen in all people with the diagnosis, certain characteristics are commonly associated with, and indeed frequently seen among, people diagnosed with Asperger Syndrome.

These include the following:

- **Highly intelligent and often intellectual:** Many people with AS excel in school and have many academic interests. Others are very bright but do not do so well within the school environment. Most have average intelligence, and many have above-average learning ability.

- **Tendency to be socially awkward and to lack awareness of social conventions:** Many adults with AS talk about not understanding the rules of social interactions. They feel at a loss in social situations, often making mistakes or not knowing what to do or say. Some have compared it to feeling like "aliens" on a strange new planet where they don't understand what is expected or how to behave.

- **Black-and-white thinking:** Frequently literal and concrete thinkers, many people with AS exhibit a tendency to view things in extremes (e.g., all or nothing, right or wrong, good or bad). They struggle to perceive the gradations, the "gray" areas.

- **Inflexibility:** Shifting gears, tolerating interruptions, incorporating feedback or responding to others' perceptions is extremely challenging for the AS adult.

- **Difficulty with change, transitions:** Related to inflexibility, AS adults can become "stuck" or hyper-focused. They may find it hard to tolerate changes in routine and to move smoothly from one situation or activity to another.

- **"Theory of mind" challenges:** This relates to the ability to envision another's point of view. People with AS often assume that others view the world as they do, rather than with their own perspectives and viewpoints. They also tend to miss the nonverbal cues that might guide them to see that this is most often not the case. For example, they might not notice that someone is bored with hearing about the special interest they are talking about – they don't tune in to the listener's yawns, roaming eyes, or other signals that indicate that the other person is not as interested in this topic as the speaker.

- **Organizational and attentional difficulties:** People with AS almost universally report difficulties with time management and organizational skills (establishing and maintaining a routine, meeting deadlines, being on time for appointments, forgetting, losing things, etc.). Rooms and book bags are stuffed – things can't be found. In terms of attention, many experience difficulty staying focused, often drifting into fantasizing or surreptitiously reading. On the other hand, given a pleasurable activity such as reading or working/playing on the computer, they may become over-focused and be unable to break away.

- **Sensory integration issues:** Many people with AS have limited tolerance or heightened sensitivity to sounds, smells, touch. They become easily overwhelmed, become confused with too much stimulation of any sort (visual, crowds). May experience extreme discomfort relative to temperature and clothing, called "tactile defensiveness."

Understanding Your Profile

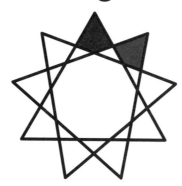

The key to success is to understand your own personal profile and to convert that awareness into plans, strategies and interventions to achieve your goals. Because these plans are customized to reflect your specific needs and goals, and because you will be participating in developing them yourself, they are more likely to be successful.

Typical Goals/Atypical Mind

Individuals on the spectrum tend to develop at a different rate than their neurotypical peers. Despite their average to superior intelligence, they do not notice things in the world around them and exhibit significant delays in many areas. Frequently there are delays in the development of independent life skills such as

- the use of money,
- management of time,
- organizational skills,
- performance of tasks of daily living, and
- social relationships.

Such delays in the development of independent life skills (ILS) may significantly hinder the ability to separate from family, to become independent, to go off to college or to live on one's own.

Here's an opportunity to check your progress in the development of these important skills.

What's Your Independent Life Skills Timetable?

Developmental History

The growth and development of young children is measured by so-called developmental milestones, such as age of first tooth, first steps, first words, and so on. Although we do not call them milestones, there are also benchmarks of development throughout adolescence and adulthood. Puberty is the most obvious example. But there are other "markers": first date, first kiss, first apartment, first job, etc.

Underlying these important steps are the independent life skills that enable the young person to reach these milestones. For example, generally, you can't have a first date if you can't cross the street by yourself. You can't get a job if you won't put on clean clothes for an interview. These are the "givens," the unspoken markers of maturity and readiness for independence.

What are the expectations for someone your age?
What is typical of the neurotypical adolescent or adult?

A way to find out is to ask or observe people around you and compare their skills to yours. Another way is to look at life skills assessment tools, many of which may be located on the web. These assessment tools give you an idea of the skills that are expected of an emerging adult (roughly age 16 and up). I have included several samples of these types of assessment tools in the Appendix. These can be pretty intimidating to complete, but they give you an idea of what skills are assumed to be developed by a certain age.

As mentioned above, Asperger Syndrome is considered a pervasive developmental disorder and, as such, implies that there is a delay in the development of certain skills. Thus, it is likely that there is a gap between the skill development of the neurotypical and your development of these skills.

Have you noticed some specific areas that need
further development?

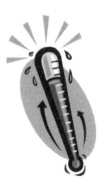

Areas in Need of Further Development

Record some of your perceptions here.

I notice that most people my age are able to:

☐ Live on their own _____

☐ Keep track of belongings _____

☐ Get to appointments on time and on their own _____

☐ Keep their room or home organized _____

☐ Pay bills _____

Other examples:

I notice that I am not yet able to:

_____

_____

I have pretty good skills in: (check those that apply and give some examples)

☐ Money management: _____

☐ Time management: _____

☐ Organization: _____

Independent Life Skills (ILS) – a.k.a. Tasks of Daily Living (TDL):

☐ Basic hygiene: _____

☐ Managing own medicine: _____

☐ Managing time: _____

☐ Social relationships: _____

☐ I still need to develop my skills in: _____

Later on in this workbook, you will be able to do a more extensive and more specific evaluation of your progress in developing independent life skills. In the meantime, this exercise may have helped you begin to appreciate that you have your own developmental timetable that is likely somewhat different from that of your neurotypical age-mates.

A classic example of the unique timetable of people on the spectrum occurs in mid to late adolescence. Just when most young adults are individuating and separating from their parents, are getting ready to move away from home, be more independent, etc., many young people with spectrum disorders continue to need significant support and monitoring due to challenges in judgment, common sense, and life skills.

Despite such challenges and delays, adolescents and adults with AS and related disorders want pretty much the same things that everyone else wants, even if they don't understand exactly why. For example, they might want friends, but express confusion about what people get out of a relationship or what's enjoyable about being with other people. They may feel isolated, yet they are uncomfortable around people.

To make these goals more attainable, you must identify the gaps in "mainstream" skills – basic life and communication skills – and make accommodations and adjustments so you will be able to make optimal use of your superior intellect.

In this workbook you will have the opportunity to do this. You will be asked to:

- set goals
- determine the skills necessary to reach your goals
- realistically assess what you need to be able to do to get to where you want to be
- make a plan for achieving those self-set goals.

So – let's get started.

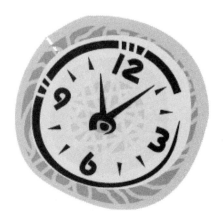

Your Vision and Goals:
Vision – Goal – Plan (VGP)

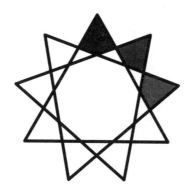

The process for enhancing the quality of your life starts with a vision and a set of goals. What do you want for yourself – in the short term and in the future? Here's the sequence we will follow:

1. Create a Vision
2. Identify Your Goals
3. Assess Your Skills
4. Set Priorities
5. Target the Areas Needing Growth
6. Close the Gaps

Create a Vision

This is your chance to explore your potential and your dreams. A *vision* is a portrait of what you would like to see in your life within a defined time frame. It's a "snapshot" or picture of what you hope your life will be like. It's fantasy but with a reality base. Although we all might like to be multi-gazillionaires, married to royalty or living in space, a true vision needs to be attainable and realistic. For example, my vision for retirement is to travel with my family as much as possible, to give talks, and to spend more months out of the year in a warm climate.

Think big and "out of the box," but not off the planet! Some examples might be: to own your own home and have a job in a library; or to be married and living in the country rather than the city.

Your *goals* are derived from your vision. They are the things you must do to create the life you have envisioned – that is, to reach your vision. For example, if you have a partner or significant other in your vision, your goals might include learning how to have more intimate relationships, or learning how to live with others. If you would like meaningful work, you may have to acquire better interview skills; if you want to have friends, you may need to master a bit of the art of small talk (and have a certain level of "cultural literacy").

My Vision

Don't Give up Your Dreams!

1. Where would you like to see yourself in five years?

   _____

   _____

   _____

2. In ten years?

   _____

   _____

   _____

3. Describe the life you envision in as much detail as possible.

   Where do you live? _____

   What kind of home? _____

   What is your job? _____

   Who do you live with? _____

   What do you do for fun? _____

   What is a typical day like? _____

   What is a typical week like? _____

Write a brief description of your imagined life:

_____

_____

_____

_____

_____

_____

_____

_____

_____

You may want to create some visuals – sketches, pictures from magazines, photos. Use the space below to illustrate your vision.

You will use this vision to generate a Vision Statement (a written summary of your imagined future life) and to create goals. An example of a Vision Statement is given on the next page. Use the blank diagram to create a simplified version of your vision.

Sample Vision Statement

Vision: A fulfilling life with work and relationships goals below

1 **Meaningful work**

2 **Friends**

3 **My own apartment**

Now fill out your own.

My Personal Vision Statement

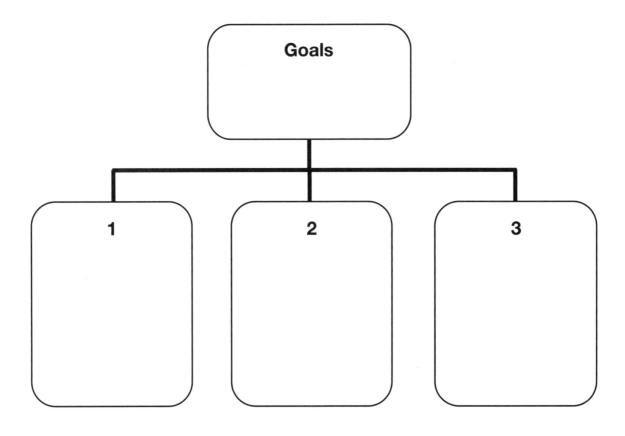

Goals

1

2

3

The goals in your Vision Statement are the steps that will bring your vision to reality.

For example, I want a job in software development; therefore, one goal might be to obtain the education, degree or credentials needed to obtain such a position. Check the *Occupational Outlook Handbook* to determine the specific requirements for the type of work you are considering. The *Occupational Outlook Handbook* may be obtained from your local library or perused on-line (http://www.bls.gov/oco). It includes descriptions of most occupations and careers, including qualifications, projected opportunities in the future and related occupations. It is useful in broadening awareness of career options as well as providing information about how to prepare for obtaining each type of employment.

There is no glass ceiling – no limit to what a person with AS can achieve. Most of what does not come intuitively or naturally can be acquired or learned. What is mechanical, contrived or even robotic at first can become quite natural with time and practice. For example, there are many ways to greet someone – verbally ("hello," "hi," "what's up?") and nonverbally (nod, wave, wink). Individuals with AS frequently utilize only one type of greeting in all situations. However, if they learn several different greetings for various circumstances and practice them in advance, their greetings will become more fluid, more appropriate to the circumstance and more natural.

Hold on to your dreams and don't give up trying to attain your goals.

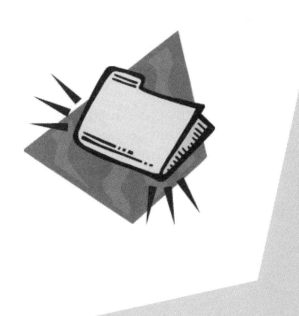

Identify Your Goals

The first step is to identify your goals. Using your vision, identify goals and list them in priority order.

These are some of the things I would need to accomplish in order to have the kind of life I have envisioned:

1. _____

2. _____

3. _____

4. _____

5. _____

Examples:

- Meaningful, enjoyable job in an area of interest and at a level commensurate with my skills, background and experience
- Circle of friends
- Love relationship
- My own home

An Example

In 1994 I met Michelle. A recent graduate of a prestigious women's college, Michelle had been diagnosed with Asperger Syndrome a short while earlier. Despite communication, organizational, social and spatial challenges, Michelle had some very clear goals. She wanted "a life," which to her meant meaningful work, friends, a love relationship, enjoyable recreational activities, a home of her own and independence. She had a clear vision and was determined to achieve her goals. Through hard work, Michelle has achieved all of her goals.

Today she is employed (having obtained a master's degree), has moved to the northwest with her husband, has friends, and enjoys a wide range of activities, including tai chi, motorcycle riding, outdoor hiking, canoeing and Toastmasters. She is active in the local Asperger support network and has spoken at conferences about her experiences.

Michelle is one example of what can be achieved, given a vision and set of goals. Although not everyone will be as successful as Michelle has been, a vision provides a direction, and everyone should be able to move some distance along that path.

Things to Consider as You Set Goals

People with AS frequently find themselves unemployed or under-employed (working at a job for which they are considerably overqualified). Despite average to above-average intelligence, and frequently exceptional academic credentials, weaknesses in the "presentation of self" prevent many AS adults from obtaining a position in their field of expertise and/or at a level that is commensurate with their ability. Moreover, many adults with AS find it difficult to determine what factors would facilitate or hinder successful functioning in the workplace.

Consideration of issues such as the degree of privacy/independence versus the amount of interaction/collaboration, the pace and intensity of the environment, etc., is essential in determining the appropriateness of the position. Therefore, when setting a work goal, it is important to consider the tasks performed, the "culture" of the workplace and the "fit" to your profile.

Making a decision about what career path to choose, for example, can be approached from a variety of vantage points. Many people think of the category (for example, law, medicine, education) rather than attempting to match personal preferences with the realities of the job. As a result, people who shy away from interpersonal contact may end up preparing to become teachers, and introverts wanting to become broadcasters.

The following exercise is a way to look at what you really like to do and in what contexts. In examining these features, you can get a better idea of the "fit" with potential career choices.

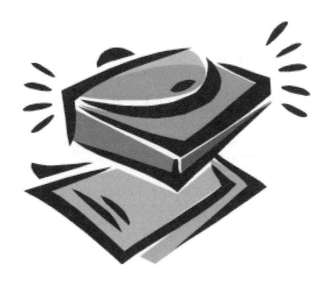

What Do I Really Like to Do and in What Contexts?

What tasks do you enjoy performing?
(example: I like to make lists; I love "surfing" the Internet; I like to read)

_____

_____

In what type of setting?
(example: large or small office, cubicle or more spacious work area, quiet work space)

_____

_____

With what degree of interaction? _____

Independent versus group work: (which do you prefer; can you handle both if necessary?)

_____

I would like to work alone_____

☐ I would like to work on my own most of the time but could interact for short periods (15 minutes at a time)

☐ I can envision a 50/50 split of time working independently and time working with others

☐ I am able to work near other people and can tolerate some noise and potential interruptions

☐ I like having people around me and would enjoy collaborating with others

And with how much stress? (*example: busy, bustling office or retail store, hectic pace, frequent deadlines, unpredictable changes*)

_____

_____

_____

Deadlines (Can you meet them?)

☐ Yes

☐ No

Use of Telephone

☐ I would prefer not to have to use the telephone.

☐ I am able to use the telephone when I have sufficient time to think about what I say.

☐ I am totally comfortable answering the telephone and/or making calls.

Socialization

☐ I would prefer to be by myself during work hours.
☐ I would take a coffee or lunch break with my coworker(s).
☐ I would like to get to know my colleague(s).
☐ I would like to have friends at work.
☐ I would like to do social activities with colleagues.

Sensory Considerations

Work space/environment – Is there enough light? Too much? Enough space or close quarters? Distractions? Noise?

_____

_____

_____

Opportunities for sensory breaks (quiet space)

_____

_____

_____

Other:

_____

_____

_____

_____

_____

Now use the information you generated above to describe your "ideal" work setting:

_____

_____

_____

_____

_____

_____

_____

_____

Set realistic and appropriate goals by acknowledging and respecting your profile, your talents and your comfort zone.

Other Ways to Explore Your Career Options

There are many career assessment tools available in print, on the Web, as well as through employment agencies, career counselors and vocational services. You may want to compare your results to the results you get from completing one of these more "formal" assessments. An example of a formal assessment is included in the Appendix. An excellent online resource is www.O-Net.com.

Assessment

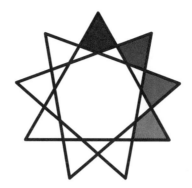

How Prepared Are You to Pursue Your Goals?

Now look at the specific behaviors you already exhibit or are likely to exhibit that may impact your performance in the job(s) you are considering, or the goals you hope to achieve.

Are you able to distinguish which behaviors might help you perform the job or attain a goal you have set? Can you tell what behaviors might be hindrances?

Think about your goals and the things you do or could do to enable you to move forward towards achievement. These questions may help you refine your thinking about how to go about working toward your goals:

1. Behaviors that are likely to **facilitate** achievement of: (select one of your goals to do this exercise)
   (*example: if one of your goals is to live on your own, a facilitating behavior would be saving up some money; if you hope to be a bank teller, a facilitating behavior is accurate calculating*)

   _____

   _____

   _____

2. Behaviors that are likely to **hinder** achievement of your goal: (*example: using all your money to buy video games when you are saving up for something; or extreme shyness when you are hoping to be a politician*)

   _____

   _____

   _____

3. Plans for implementing facilitating behaviors: *(example: ask a trusted ally to keep your bankbook for you – carry a single check instead of the whole checkbook)*

_____

_____

_____

_____

_____

4. Plans for eliminating or minimizing hindrances: *(example: putting your ATM or credit card in a lockbox so they are not so easy to get to; creating a budget; avoiding going into stores with video games, etc.)*

_____

_____

_____

_____

_____

You may need some help to come up with these strategies. Consult other Aspies or people who work well with people on the spectrum.

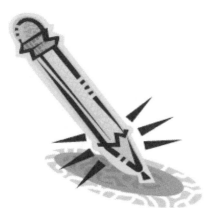

26

Independent Life Skills – A Reality Checklist

Now that you've identified your goals, the next step is to honestly appraise what could be or might be getting in the way of achieving them. Start with a Life Skills Assessment (see page 29). It might hurt to look at yourself this way, but it will help you figure out what skills you need to develop as well as areas where you are quite accomplished and do well.

As part of this activity, please read and think about the following statement:

Not everything that is faced can be changed,
but nothing can be changed until it is faced.
– Source unknown

What does this statement mean to you?

_____

_____

_____

Can you think of things you haven't wanted to face? If so, what?

_____

_____

Are you ready to face these things now? _____

Why? _____

_____

What makes it possible for you to do this now? _____

_____

_____

Now this one is really hard:

What have others told you repeatedly that you have denied or rejected? *(example: your parents, teachers, employers make suggestions about how to keep track of things because you frequently misplace things, yet you insist that there isn't a problem and that you have a workable system; another example: you have been told over and over that your voice volume is too high; you are offended and feel you have the right to talk as loudly as you wish.)*

_____

_____

_____

_____

_____

Are they correct? Why or why not?

_____

_____

_____

_____

_____

You have the potential to do most anything, but may be hindered by "small" but significant skill deficits. For example, you might have the credentials for admission to a great college or getting a wonderful job, but you can't get yourself up in the morning independently.

Be honest as you fill this out. As a reality check, you might ask an "impartial" person to also fill out a checklist so that you can compare your perceptions to those of someone else who knows you well.

Keep your goals in mind – and remember: You can't achieve them if you don't address the constraints.

Independent Life Skills Assessment

OK ... you feel ready to move ahead towards achieving your goals. A next step is to assess the degree to which you have developed the skills you will need. That is, determine what skills you need to do what you'd like to do and to what extent you have developed those skills.

As promised, here is your chance to do a more specific evaluation of the level of your independent life skills. This Independent Life Skills Assessment tool can help you determine any gaps that need to be addressed. It differs from the assessments you have already begun in two ways: (1) it can be easily compared with (an)other's perception and (2) it breaks the skills down into very basic and specific areas, many of which are common problem areas for people on the spectrum.

Independent Life Skills Assessment

Instructions: This checklist is a self-evaluation. Check the appropriate box based on how often you perform the task independently, with no guidance or prompting. To obtain the best, most comprehensive profile, also have this checklist completed by parent(s), teacher(s) or any other helping adult who knows you well. This will give you some basis for comparison between your perceptions and the way you are perceived by others.

	Always	Frequently	Occasionally	Rarely	Never
Gets up on own					
Washes					
Showers					
Brushes teeth					
Combs hair					
Wears clean clothes					
Eats					
Takes medicines					
Seeks medical care					
Dresses appropriately for weather conditions					
Able to remember basic tasks/messages					
Keeps track of belongings					
Able to drive or take public transportation					
Able to get to destination on time					
ACADEMIC FUNCTIONING					
Records assignments					
Completes assignments					
Hands in assignments					
On time with virtually no assistance					
May require accommodations but not monitoring/prodding					
Is aware of some learning needs					
Able to advocate for self or obtain an advocate					
Able to follow academic rules (read what is assigned, show work, etc.)					
Will follow teacher instruction					
COMMUNICATION SKILLS					
Uses appropriate greetings with eye contact (no staring or lack of eye contact)					
Able and willing to communicate needs and questions					
Affect matches circumstance/topic/situation					
Able to control: • Obsessions					
• Self-stimulation					
• Inappropriate responses/meltdowns until in a private location or as prearranged with helping adults					
Able to engage in "small talk" for short periods					
Able to: • Begin conversations					
• Sustain conversations					
• Terminate conversation					
RELATIONSHIPS					
Able to engage with helping adults other than parents					
Aware of others to extent that actions and behaviors do not adversely affect them					
Understands the basics of relationships, such as levels and associated rules, the concept of reciprocity, etc.					

Additional Information

If there are basic life skills that you feel are important but that are not listed on page 30, please add them here and note your level of mastery. (*example: able to wait turn in conversation; able to respond to previous remarks and statements rather than going off on own tangent*)

_____

_____

_____

_____

_____

_____

_____

_____

_____

_____

_____

_____

As you examine your results, sort the skills and record them as follows on page 32. If all evaluators (yourself and anybody else you have asked to also complete the checklist) chose "always" for a skill, list that as a "solid skill"; if there is difference of opinion or not all checked "always," list the skill under "needs some work." If all or most evaluators checked "occasionally," "rarely" or "never," such skills are "underdeveloped."

Life Skills Assessment Summary and Timetable

Skill	Needs Some Work	Underdeveloped	Priority	Next Steps/Timetable

If you've filled this out honestly to the best of your knowledge and/or have compared your results with those of an "objective ally," you should have an idea of where the gaps are in the development of your independent living skills, or ILS. For example, if one of your goals is to live in your own home, but you can't drive or take public transportation, can't cook, or can't get up in the morning on your own, you can see that you have some work to do to reach your goal.

As you develop a plan for "closing the gaps," you will use the data you have generated to set priorities. For example, if a skill is basic, it must be addressed first ... like brushing your teeth! Or if a skill is essential to your biggest goal, you need to work on it first.

This is the beginning of the process of identifying the skills you need to address as well as the timetable for addressing them. What are your priorities? Be sure to check them on your Life Skills Assessment Summary and Timetable.

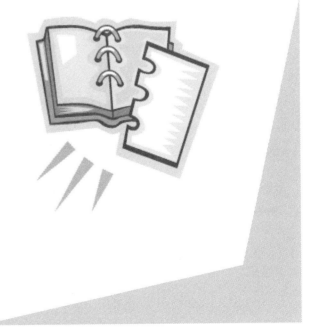

Self-Appraisal

A profile is not only about constraints and weaknesses. As mentioned earlier, you have many strong suits to bring to bear. Strengths, preferences, etc., are also part of the picture. Use this chart to flesh out your profile.

Personal Profile

Strengths *(example: good reader)*	**Weaknesses** *(example: math)*
Things I Love *(example: reading, chocolate)*	**Things I Hate** *(example: housework)*
Things That Disturb Me *(make me feel uncomfortable, such as spiders, skull & crossbones)*	**Things That Soothe Me** *(example: my satin pillowcase)*

Note: Things that are *disturbing* to you make you feel "icky" like moldy bathrooms or "haunted houses." *Feeling anxious*, on the other hand, is more of an ongoing or repeating rather than transitory experience (new situations, elevators). Of course, these are quite similar experiences for some people, and frequently things that are disturbing may make you anxious. For example, I am disturbed by spiders and, as a result, if I see one, I become anxious and worry that there may be more of them around.

There are many ways to develop your profile. You can use a pre-developed checklist such as the one above, or you can challenge yourself to identify characteristics that operate as facilitators or as constraints in your life.

Most older adolescents and adults with AS are well aware of the things that get in their way even if they don't generally admit it. Now's the time to acknowledge the constraints so you can address them. You might as well; you've already bought this book and filled out some of it, so you can't return it. Seriously, the more you know about your profile, the more you will be able to exercise some control over impediments and obstacles OR, better yet, the more you will be able to take advantage of your assets – see below. It's like the old saying, "It's what you don't know that will hurt you." Anyway, you don't have to show this to anyone else!

Compare Yourself to the "Classic Profile" of Individuals with Asperger Syndrome

Refer back to the list of common characteristics at the beginning of the book and below to begin to compare your own profile with the "classic" profile. These are some of the common areas of concern expressed by adults with AS:

- Time management

- Organization

- Flexibility

- Communication

- Awareness of others and the world around them

- Sensory issues

- Anxiety

Here's your chance to put your concerns "on the table." Be as specific as you can – it will help you figure out how to intervene as part of the process of achieving your goals.

Examples might be "I am forgetful and miss appointments," "I sometimes forget to shower or don't leave enough time to shower before I have to go out," "People don't seem to like me; when I was younger people teased me a lot."

Results of Self-Appraisal

I notice that I have trouble with:

1. _____

2. _____

3. _____

4. _____

5. _____

6. _____

7. _____

8. _____

9. _____

10. _____

Whew! What a process! By now you have looked at your functioning in several different ways and have generated a good deal of information about what you do well and what skills or areas need development. Ideally, these exercises have helped you refine your thinking about what you hope to accomplish (your vision and goals). Hopefully, you have also begun to identify (acknowledge) underdeveloped skills.

This next section will guide you in a process of setting priorities (what areas to target first) as well as how to begin to address the constraints you have identified, what areas you need to work on and what areas you want to target first.

PART 2: PUTTING IT ALL TOGETHER

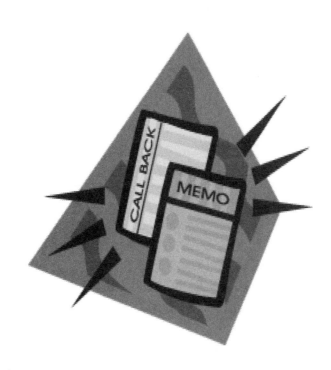

From Profile to Plan

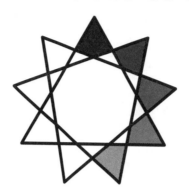

Take a few moments to congratulate yourself on getting this far. Look over your work and try to be a "camera." "Zoom out" to get a view of the whole you, a complex and unique combination of strengths and weaknesses, preferences and challenges. Then "zoom in" to identify the areas needing work in developing independent life skills, relationships, leisure activities and dating, and acquiring and maintaining employment.

The next step in this process is to use the information you have generated to formulate a plan. The graphic below summarizes the process we have been discussing: a pathway to independence, or to achieving the goals you have set.

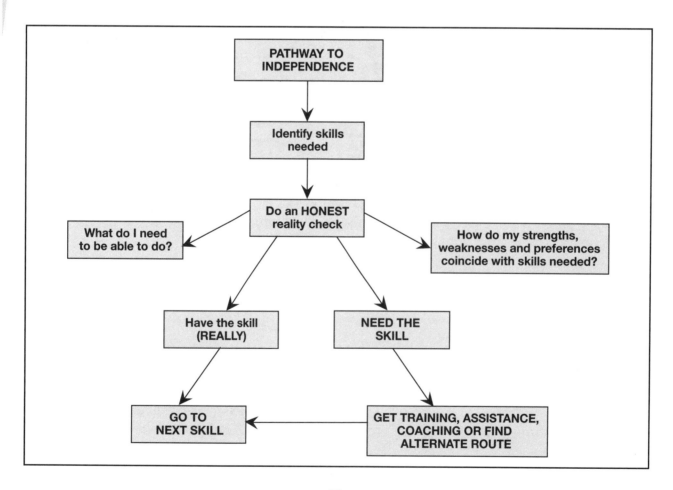

Here is what this looks like using a specific skill such as time management.

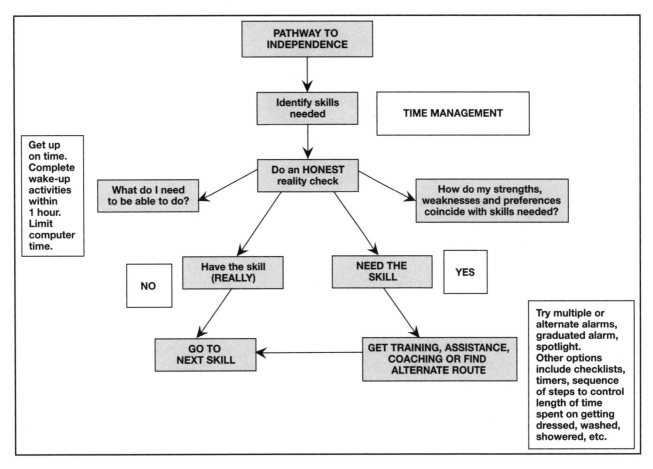

If you are nonvisual and are wondering, "what's all that?" here's the translation of the visual above summarizing the process we have outlined:

1. Identify the skills necessary to accomplish one of your goals (such as better time management).
2. Do an honest appraisal of what you need to be able to do *and* to what degree you are able to do it.
3. Utilizing resources if available and appropriate, develop and try out techniques and strategies until you find what works for you.
4. When satisfied, move on to the next needed skill.

So, where are we?

We've ...

- identified a vision,
- set some goals,
- and determined some of the skills you will need. (Refer to your Life Skills Assessment Summary and Timetable as well as the results of your Self-Appraisal.)

Now it's time to begin working on developing your skills.

Coaching

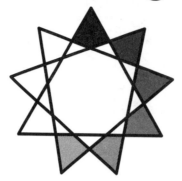

As you continue working on or developing your skills relative to your vision and goals, you will need some help. You may work with a friend or a relative, or you may have a counselor or therapist you are already familiar with. An option that has proven very successful is to find a "coach," not in the traditional sports sense but as outlined below.

Why Coaching?

Why choose coaching over other forms of treatment, counseling or therapy? Coaching is best seen as an adjunct or add-on service rather than a sole solution. That is, coaching works best when it is part of an array of services, which may include psychiatry, psychopharmacology (medication management and monitoring), psychotherapy (the treatment of mental disorders by psychological methods), vocational counseling, etc.

Coaching differs from other types of support in several aspects. It is not therapy in the traditional sense, although it is therapeutic by virtue of the progress made by the participant. It is a team approach. It is directive and practical. Goals are identified and analyzed relative to factors that have interfered with attainment of goals. These factors are then systematically targeted for interventions that may eliminate or at least neutralize their influence.

Let's look at some examples:

Goal	Hindrance	Intervention
• Obtain job	• Come to job interview in messy clothes, sandals, uncombed hair	• Notice what others wear, ask for help to create more traditional appearance
• Make a friend	• Avoid eye contact, not know name	• Greet by name with eye contact

This model requires an ability to identify "neurotypical" behavior and to compare it to your own current behavior. It requires some ability to observe others as well as to recognize and acknowledge problem areas.

The coach does not act as an "expert" who knows all the answers, but expects clients to figure things out for themselves. The coach does not claim to have all the answers, but sees him or herself as a partner in a collaborative effort for the purpose of solving problems. The process is simple: The client identifies goals; the client and coach collaborate to identify factors that have interfered in the past; priorities are set for targeting interferences; the coach makes suggestions for strategies, which the client then tries out; progress is monitored; and interventions are evaluated and refined as needed. In short, coaching is simply a process of the client saying what s/he wants and the coach helping him/her figure out what to do to get it.

Coaching in a Nutshell

Coaching: A collegial relationship focusing on personal goals, offering practical ideas and strategies for improving functioning in all areas of life, including

- Job
- School
- Social skills
- Organizational skills
- Life skills

What it is ...

- Therapeutic but not psychotherapy
- Focused on the here and now and on the future
- Concrete and practical
- Directive
- Pragmatic problem-solving approach
- Metacognitive – knowledge about your own thoughts and the factors that influence your thinking (from *Encarta Online Dictionary*)
- Collegial – a sharing of knowledge and insight between equals

What it's not ...

- Psychotherapy
- Focused on the past
- Concerned with others' role in the cause or solution to problems
- A relationship between an "expert" who withholds insights and a "patient" who must discover what the expert already knows

You and Coaching

Now that you know a little bit about coaching, what do you think? Is it something you can see yourself getting involved in?

Many folks prefer the coaching approach because they can set the agenda themselves. In addition, the focus is on the concerns and wishes you come up with yourself rather than problems identified by others. In other words, it's an "I'd like to do better at ..." approach versus "You should be able to ..." approach.

You may be able to locate a coach through your local Asperger's association, parent's group, or from a teacher or counselor. Local psychiatrists, psychologists, social workers or mental health personnel may also know of coaches in your area. Finally, an Internet search for "autism" or "Asperger's" coach may be fruitful.

Getting Started

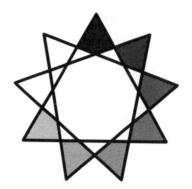

Set Priorities

Begin at the beginning and develop a logical sequence of steps.

What can you target first? How about:

- Awakening on your own?
- Daily self-care and hygiene?

In choosing where and how to begin, be sure to distinguish between what is a *problem* versus what is a *preference* For example, with regard to hair care, it may be your preference to have longish hair, but it's a problem if it's unkempt, dirty, dangerous on the job, etc. Similarly, with regard to selection of clothes, you may prefer a particular style. This only becomes a problem if it is wildly inappropriate for the setting (formal gown to go bowling, jeans at a formal wedding) or dirty, torn, poor condition, blatantly mismatched.

> **Tip:** Use observation, of or corroboration from, neurotypicals to determine how often you get a haircut, if you should shave daily, etc.

Steps to Prioritizing

1. Pick out some people in each "section" of your life (work, school, neighborhood, church/synagogue) who seem to be "popular," well liked, well respected, successful, satisfied and self-confident.

   List their names here:

   _____

   _____

   _____

2. Now observe them (be discreet and subtle) and notice what they do, how they look, how they act and, if possible, what they say.

   What words would you use to describe them? What do others say about them?

   List the words – write the meanings and identify a specific behavior you could use to demonstrate this quality.

Word	Meaning	Specific Action
"clean-cut"	neat and clean	wash, comb hair
friendly	nice to others	make eye contact/smile

3. Can you think of additional descriptors you can add to the list:

   _____

   _____

   _____

   _____

4. Next, evaluate your behaviors relative to the people you have observed.

   For example: S/he greets people by name with a smile and eye contact, whereas I look down when I pass someone I know, so I don't have to greet them.

   Can you identify some other comparisons/contrasts between your behavior and the behavior of the "successful" people you have observed:

   _____

   _____

   _____

   _____

   _____

Has this helped you figure out some areas to work on? If not,

- Get some help from a trusted ally to check your accuracy in observing or comparing
  Or
- Go through the process again: identify observable behaviors of "successful" neurotypicals and compare them with your behavior. If you cannot do this alone, get help!

Create a Plan

5. Now list the most important areas to work on and the order in which you will address them:

a. _____

b. _____

c. _____

d. _____

e. _____

f. _____

6. Now that you've figured out which areas to work on, find the "entry point" and steps for working on your first skill.

   For example, getting up in the morning on your own.
   Where can you start; what can you adjust in order to help you do this?

   Step 1: What am I currently doing?

   _____

   Step 2: What can I try instead?

   _____

   Example: Set a reasonable bedtime/wake-up time, given your current pattern. Can you go to bed an hour earlier and get up an hour earlier? A half hour? Do you need an alarm? Two alarms? How about putting a timer on a bright light that will shine in your face at a preset time? How about an automatic computer shutdown so you can go to sleep? Some students at Massachusetts Institute of Technology (MIT) have developed an alarm clock, called Clocky, that has to be chased around the room in order to be able to shut it off. Try one if you have difficulties in this area.

My Plan for Getting up on My Own in the Morning

_____

_____

_____

_____

_____

_____

_____

_____

_____

Follow this process of identifying the "entry" point and breaking down each skill you target. Get ideas from others or from the coach, if you have one.

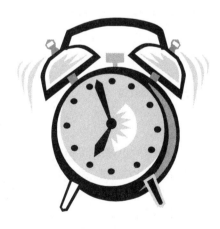

Break Tasks Down into Small, Doable Steps

An important component of this process is to work systematically in small increments, building success upon success rather than attempting too much at one time. It is advisable to create a logical sequence of skills to target (prioritize) and then break them down into steps.

Example:

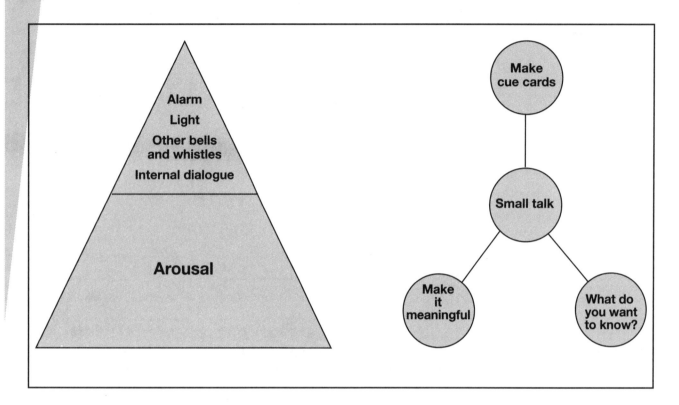

Congratulations!

You've come a long way, and by now you should have

- Your vision
- Your goals
- Your areas needing attention
- The beginnings of a plan

And for our visual learners, here's what that might look like:

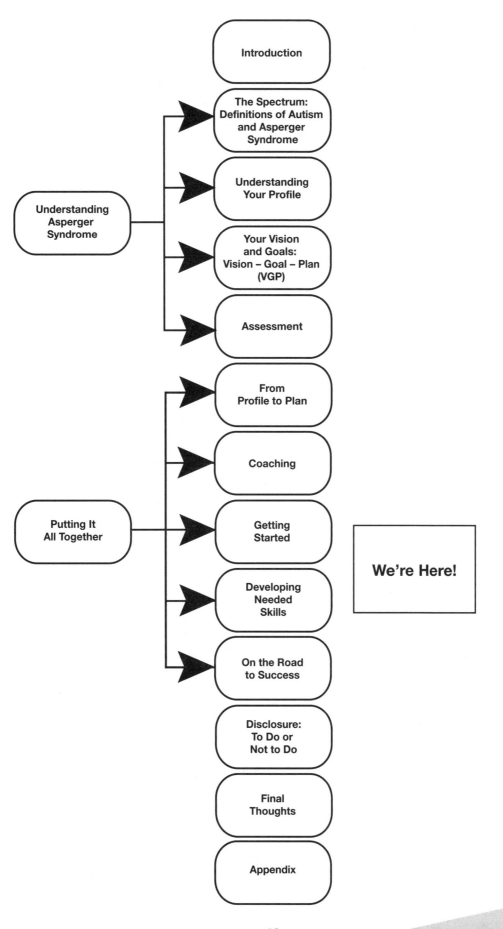

Introduction

The Spectrum:
Definitions of Autism
and Asperger
Syndrome

Understanding
Your Profile

Understanding
Asperger
Syndrome

Your Vision
and Goals:
Vision – Goal – Plan
(VGP)

Assessment

From
Profile to Plan

Coaching

Putting It
All Together

Getting
Started

We're Here!

Developing
Needed
Skills

On the Road
to Success

Disclosure:
To Do or
Not to Do

Final
Thoughts

Appendix

Developing Needed Skills

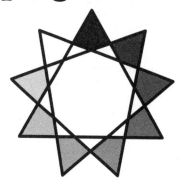

Now the best part! This section offers a host of ideas and strategies to try out to improve your quality of life. The areas selected as examples illustrate how very basic the skills are that need to be addressed by people with autism spectrum disorders. Things that seem obvious to the neurotypical often elude the person with AS. Just saying "hello" when you meet a coworker in the hallway can be a challenge. These examples also represent some of the most common areas of concern for adults on the spectrum who are attempting to become more independent.

These strategies are offered here because they have been used successfully by others and are seen as some of the best practices available. Some will work for you, some may not, but they will help you refine the process of developing alternatives to problematic behaviors. Zosia Zaks's exceptional book *Life and Love: Positive Strategies for Autistic Adults* published by the Autism Asperger Publishing Company (www.asperger.net) is another excellent source of information on strategies and accommodations.

Strategies

Developing strategies is an ongoing process. New circumstances and situations arise all the time. You need a method for analyzing the situation, obtaining any needed information and creating an appropriate way to handle the situation.

Many people don't have a clear procedure for doing this.

One technique that has proven effective for people on the spectrum is to consult or observe neurotypical age-mates and to view models of what is appropriate in various situations. The process is simple and covers a broad range of situations. You can use it to decide what to wear, what to bring to someone's house when invited to dinner and how to act at all kinds of social situations (from wedding to funerals).

Many of these situations are fraught with "unwritten rules," things people assume everyone knows but that elude the person with AS. Observing neurotypicals or consulting books such as *The Hidden Curriculum – Practical Solutions for Understanding Unstated Rules in Social*

Situations by Brenda Smith Myles, Melissa Trautman, and Ronda Schelvan (www.asperger.net) can yield invaluable information about what to do or how to act.

The following simple chart may help.

Situation	Rules – Written and Unwritten	Observations	Protocol
Guest at wedding	Don't wear white		Respond to invitation by due date; buy or send present; dress appropriately
Best man at wedding	Give a toast		Write out what you will say
Services in place of worship	Wear a head covering? Wear dress clothes (no pants for women)		Be sure to wear appropriate clothing

It is important to know what is expected in unfamiliar situations where you don't know the rules or traditions. For example, in some houses of worship, it is forbidden for women to wear pants or to leave your head uncovered. You may want to consult someone you know who is of that faith to be sure what to do if you have occasion to visit. If you don't know any-one, try the Internet or books on religious customs.

Many people with AS report that they have inadvertently insulted someone because they did not know how to act in certain situations. To avoid this, prepare for unfamiliar situations by obtaining information from etiquette books, people you know or any other source of accurate information. Don't be afraid to ask.

PAPI Model

The PAPI model is a powerful protocol you can use for preparing for new situations and experiences. Again, it may be used in a wide range of situations, from very simple to more complex. It is comprised of four steps:

- **P**redict
- **A**nticipate
- **P**lan
- **I**mplement

Step One: Predict

What is likely to happen? To be said? What questions might be asked? What can I expect? Example: In a job interview, the interviewer is not likely to ask what you ate for lunch but is likely to ask why you want the job.

Step Two: Anticipate

What do I need to do to prepare for this? What information do I need? What skills?

Step Three: Plan

Develop a plan for obtaining information and/or skills needed for getting prepared.

Step Four: Implement

Follow through with your plan.

To illustrate, let's use PAPI in preparing to transition to independent living.

Predict:

New tasks I will need to perform:

- Shopping
- Cooking
- Transportation
- Bill paying
- Self-care

Concrete differences I should expect, such as:

- Lots of unsupervised time (will you get lost on the computer?)
- No one to remind you of things
- More solitary time
- Responsible for own food, medicine, etc.

Anticipate:

- I will need to learn simple cooking
- I will need to make a schedule so I remember to do chores, take my medicine, etc.
- I need to take a driving course

Prepare: Begin the process of obtaining the skills needed, starting by breaking skills down into small steps (e.g., get your learner's permit, then arrange for driving lessons). Identify potential allies, resources, friends, or neighbors you can develop a relationship with in order to avoid isolation.

Implement: Follow your plan to acquire skills; evaluate and revise your plan as needed or move to the next skill identified on your Life Skills Assessment Summary and Timetable.

We will be using PAPI to prepare for several common situations: change from one school level to the next, job interview or new job. It is a useful tool for a variety of circumstances and situations from field trips, to family travel, to new experiences such as the opera or a Bar Mitzvah, or to more mundane situations such as going to a movie. It is reassuring when you have thought through:

- What is likely to occur?
- What do I need to do to prepare?
  and
- You have done what was needed to be able to manage.

Using the PAPI
(Predict, Anticipate, Prepare and Implement) Rubric

A blank template is given below for you to try to utilize the PAPI model to prepare for a new situation.

Now try it out. Fill out a PAPI sequence for a situation you may be anticipating.

What's the new situation: _____

Predict (What is likely to occur?):

_____

_____

_____

Anticipate (What do you need to know or do to prepare?):

_____

_____

_____

Prepare (What steps can you take to get ready?):

_____

_____

_____

Implement: Do It!!

Managing Transitions and New Situations

Adolescents and adults with AS often have great difficulty with transitions and new situations. They tend to have limited ability to anticipate, predict and intuit, with a generalized lack of understanding of social rules or norms. Moreover, they tend to be perseverative and obsessive – they rely on routine and are comforted by the familiar.

As a result, they may:

- experience change as stressful and noxious
- become anxious or inflexible, especially if changes are unexpected

For these reasons, they need careful preparation and protocols in such areas as:

- transitioning from one school level to another
- transitioning to independent living
- preparing for new situations

You can **predict** that new situations you encounter will be stressful. Factors contributing to the level of stress may include:

- general anxiety about the unknown
- sensory issues related to crowds
- confusion about the hidden curriculum of social situations
- sensory issues related to physical contact (public bathrooms, dorm bathrooms/locker room, etc.)

To better manage transitions and new situations, you will need to expand your tolerance level in **preparation** for the challenges you **anticipate.** Areas that tend to be problematic include flexibility, tolerating interruptions and multitasking. Below you will find ways to do it – **implement.**

Expanding Tolerance and Flexibility

You can learn to cope with interruptions by accustoming yourself to interruptions that initially are planned and take place in a safe and private space. For example, at home you can ask someone to interrupt you at a specified time. As you become more comfortable, you can ask to be interrupted spontaneously. An excellent resource is the "call waiting" feature on telephones for planned and unplanned interruptions. With call waiting, if a call comes through while you are on the phone, you will hear a "beep"; you then must choose whether to answer the incoming call and, if so, what to do with current caller (for example, put on hold, end conversation) or to ignore the new call and finish the one you are already engaged in. A person can get pretty flustered and overwhelmed when this happens, but the more you practice quick decision making and develop some phrases you can use when this happens, the easier it will become for you to handle unexpected occurrences and interruptions.

You can "teach" yourself flexibility and multitasking by shifting attention back and forth between simultaneous activities. For example, you can watch TV and listen to a radio at the same time – shifting your attention back and forth in order to glean key information from both sources. You can read and take notes, or you can do math problems while listening to a book on tape.

There are many options for practicing shifting attention. Can you think of any you can see yourself trying?

Ways to Practice Shifting Attention

I could:

_____ and _____

_____ and _____

_____ and _____

Handling Sensory Overload

No matter how much we do to ensure that life goes smoothly, it is inevitable that some times will be more stressful than others. BE PREPARED!

Making up an emergency kit is probably one of the most important things you can do for yourself in this area. Inevitably, things will happen that will disrupt and disturb you. If you know ahead of time that you will have difficulty with a family trip, a holiday meal, an office party, dorm life, office politics, etc., make a plan for how to cope, including preparing an emergency kit. The emergency kit should be small and compact and be kept with you at all times. Include your best soothers such as a book, iPod, handheld game, gum (for sensory feedback) or candies, etc.

Your Personal Emergency Kit

What will you put in your emergency kit?

_____

_____

_____

_____

_____

What are some situations when you might need your emergency kit?

_____

_____

_____

_____

_____

What plan can you make to get to a safe, quiet place and use your kit?

_____

_____

_____

_____

_____

New Situations

An effective strategy for handling new situations (and a subset of the Prediction step of PAPI) is to preview the new situation (imagining or actually) in order to become familiar with it. For example, you may visualize the route you will need to drive (or driving it in advance when you don't have to rush).

> **Tip:** Now that GPS systems are readily available, this may be a better alternative for finding your way.

> **Tip:** Taking a tour (previewing) of a new setting is very beneficial, but creating an ally map is even better. As you tour, get to know people and attach them with various locations. Label a map of the location (new school, college, camp) with the names and pictures of these potential allies. Revisit and reconnect with allies.

More Skills to Develop/More Strategies to Learn

Communication: Greetings

You might be surprised to learn that there are many ways people greet each other, and that some ways are appropriate in some situations but not in others. Below, are listed four ways of using "hello."

   a. The Casual Hello – "How are you?" – when you wait for an answer (and possibly care)

   b. The Casual Hello – "How are you?" – when you are passing someone and don't wait for an answer – perfunctory social connection

   c. The Nonverbal Casual Hello – nod, smile, wave

   d. The "Real" Hello – "How are you?" – when you make eye contact and wait for response (and theoretically care)

See if you can match the appropriate "hello" to the following situations:

1. The bus driver on the bus you take to work: _____

2. Your boss or teacher: _____

3. You see someone you know in the supermarket, but he is several aisles down:

    _____

4. You pass a colleague or acquaintance in the hallway: _____

5. Your cousin whom you have not seen recently: _____

6. A friend you would like to know better: _____

How did you do?
(Answers: 1.b; 2.a.; 3.c.; 4.b or c; 5.d; 6.d)

If you were really off base with this exercise, be sure to read the section on relationships.

Pick out one or two greeting phrases that you feel comfortable saying, such as "What's up?"; "How's it going?" etc., for each type of greeting situation. Make sure it's age appropriate by observing others. Would an 18-year-old say "How do you do?" to a peer, or would he be more likely say "What's up"? Would a 60-year-old say "Yo, dawg"? If you are not sure, ask and observe.

> **Tip:** You may want to create cue cards for this.

Practice saying these phrases in front of a mirror. Knowing what you look like when you say something tends to give you more confidence. Because you already know how you look after doing this, you don't have to wonder or worry.

Concrete Schedules – One Day at a Time

Lack of organization is a significant problem for many people with AS. It is an area that requires you to do the "un-natural."

Many AS adolescents and adults say, "I don't _____" (fill in the blank … write down appointments, wear a watch, make a schedule or routine, etc.). Well, that may be true, but if the "natural" (what you are doing now) was working, we wouldn't be discussing this. So to change, you have to try what's not "natural." In fact, you can use what's natural to determine what might be more successful – just try the reverse or obverse, or ask neurotypical peers for suggestions and alternatives.

Example: I don't write appointments down anywhere. I just (pick one: remember them; ask my mother; rely on my mother to keep track; forget and don't show up). If you are regularly forgetting, missing or arriving late to appointments, it's pretty much a no-brainer to decide that you need a more reliable system for being on time. Choose a method to try out (electronic organizer, pocket appointment book, the planner on your cell phone, etc.) and give it a fair trial. Make a clear rule to record appointments *immediately* and do not deviate from the routine. After a trial period of a week, try another method if you choose to until you find the best NEW method that works for you.

Strategy
One technique that has been used successfully is to create a "pilot" schedule. To do so, use a template such as the one below:

- schedule all regular appointments, commitments, classes, work hours, etc.
- add regular TV shows, meal times, etc.
- also schedule worry or obsessions (see below)
- identify blocks of time available for chores; homework, relaxation
- color code, if helpful.
- post the schedule – try for one week – adjust as needed

You're probably horrified by this suggestion. You're thinking, "That's so NOT me!" Well, that may be true, but could you still be you and get to appointments (or do your chores, or meet your commitments) successfully? I'm betting that you can be on time and not forget appointments, yet still be the unique person you and others have come to know and love.

Once again, it's doing the "un-natural" when the natural is not working for you. Start out by creating a weekly schedule.

TIME	MONDAY	TUESDAY	WEDNESDAY	THURSDAY	FRIDAY	SAT/SUN
8						
9						
10						
11						
12						
1						
2						
3						
4						
5						
6						
7						
8						
9						
10						

Tip: Create cue card or schedule or put it in strategy notebook so you can take it with you. Or try using a paper planner or electronic planner to keep track of appointments, to-do lists, addresses, phone numbers, etc., that can be taken with you wherever you go.

To help get you started, take a look at the following sample schedule.

TIME	MONDAY	TUESDAY	WEDNESDAY	THURSDAY	FRIDAY	SAT/SUN
8	Breakfast	Breakfast	Breakfast	Breakfast	Breakfast	Breakfast
9	Work	Work	Work	Work	Work	Work
10						
11						
12	Lunch	Lunch	Lunch	Lunch	Lunch	Lunch
1	Worry*	Chores	Worry*	Therapy	Worry*	Therapy
2	Break	Break	Break	Break	Break	
3	Mail	Mail	Mail	Mail	Mail	Mail
4	Worry*		Coaching		Chores	Pay bills
5	Video					
6	Dinner	Dinner	Dinner	Dinner	Dinner	Dinner
7	TV		Tai Chi			
8						
9	Shower					
10						

*See page 63.

62

Managing Anxiety and Obsessions

Many people with AS have obsessions and significant anxieties. While obsessions can be a "hindrance," they frequently have meaning and serve a purpose. For example, one person's "obsession" was the Apollo 13 mission, which she later realized gave her hope for the future: If they could make it, so could she.

Obsessions are powerful and must be respected. Feelings such as anxiety do not just "go away." However, both feelings and thoughts can be contained so as to minimize their interference in successful daily functioning.

Strategy

One effective technique is to "compartmentalize;" literally, to schedule time for worry or obsessions. Scheduling such periods of time (at first, schedule generous allotments of time) may enable you to put off worrying and obsessing until the scheduled time, thereby averting the intrusion of these thoughts and behaviors throughout the day.

I tend to worry about _____

I feel anxious when I go/do _____

Something I would consider an obsession _____

To try to control these feelings and activities, I plan to _____

_____.

For example, I will schedule time for thinking and feeling. I will need_____ amount of

time and think good times during the day/week are _____

Another suggestion is to create "Worry" or "Angry" boxes where you temporarily, or permanently, "park" notes containing feelings, thoughts and ideas. Start by choosing minor worries or things that make you angry and ask yourself periodically whether you are ready to erase them from your thoughts altogether. When you are ready to eliminate them completely, you can bury the note in the ground or tear up the paper they were written on as a symbol of letting the worry or anger go. It may sound silly, but it is surprisingly liberating. Then you can move on to other worries or angers.

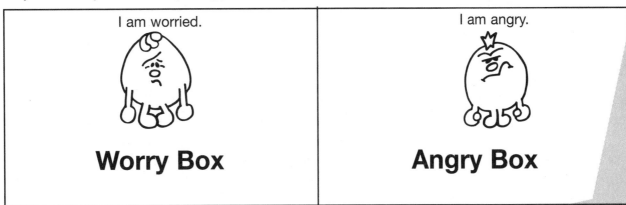

Organization: Keeping Track of Things and Controlling Clutter

Another almost universal concern among Aspies is difficulty keeping their work and living space organized and being able to find things they need. Here are some simple strategies that can help – some of them may sound ridiculously simplistic, but they work.

Strategy

1. Find a location in your space (home, office) where you will always keep certain items; for example, your keys, your glasses, your remote, your PDA, your library books, your rented videos. You can use colorful baskets or some of the great new organizing merchandise that is available. You may want to label the location.

> **Tip:** Make a firm rule that as soon as you have finished with the item, you immediately return it to its space. Never deviate from this rule.

2. Go through your mail daily (schedule this on your weekly calendar) in a location where you have set up a trash or recycle bin and/or a shredder as well as a filing system.

3. Create folders for mail to be read, mail for which action is needed and for bills. As you go through the mail, get rid of junk mail and any other materials you know you will not look at (magazines, etc. Note: if you do not read your magazines, discontinue your subscription immediately). Then sort and file the remaining mail. This can help to control the volume of paper coming in.

Strategy

To get rid of stuff you already have too much of, try this method. Take one area at a time (your desktop, bookcase, closet, etc.).

Sort according to these categories:

1. Definitely keep
2. Give away/donate
3. Return to (person, library, etc.)
4. Sell (eBay or Craigslist)
5. Throw away
6. Unsure
7. Needs action (install, download, repair)

Once you have your "piles," get rid of 2, 3 and 5. Attempt 4 for a pre-specified time (for example, list on eBay for one month. If not sold, it becomes a 2 or 5). Once these are eliminated, take care of items in 7. Locate the best place to put items you are keeping (1).

Consult an ally for items in 6 (unsure), or ask yourself a set of questions for each item you are considering getting rid of to help you make a decision:

- Do I ever use it?
- What would I use this for?
- Does it have any significance or sentimental value?
- Will I ever need it?

When done, move on to a new area and follow the same process.

Note: Although these strategies were developed by the author, other resources include similar suggestions, notably Zosia Zaks's recent book entitled *Life and Love: Positive Strategies for Autistic Adults* (www.asperger.net).

Tip: Visit www.theclutterdiet.com

Self-Care and Hygiene

Self-care and hygiene are "off the radar" for some folks with AS. I have met many people who want to go to college but don't brush their teeth; or who want to get a good job but can't get out of bed in the morning without someone hounding them; or want relationships but don't shower or use deodorant and, therefore, aren't pleasant to be close to.

Here are some ideas to try out if this is an area you struggle with, or if you have been told it is an area you need to address.

Tip: People would not say anything to you if there was not a problem – it is embarrassing for them as well as for you. So if you have been told that you have a problem, believe it and address it.

Strategy

1. Begin by determining what is "typical." As discussed previously, observation of, modeling and mentoring by neurotypical people are excellent avenues for attempting to understand and emulate "mainstream" behavior.

2. Establish a baseline for cleanliness, showering, and hand and nail care. To do so, it helps to check if your perceptions match those of others. Do you feel you are clean, but others tell you that your hair looks dirty or that you have an odor?

3. Create some rules or parameters.

   a. Define what is "clean." For example, how long should you shower? Ask trusted others for guidelines. As part of your decision-making, consider whether others may need to use the bathroom or need hot water for their showers, besides you. When is the best time for you to shower? Should you shower daily? How often should you wash your hair?

b. Determine how often to cut hair; shave; cut nails, etc. It is important to be specific here. If necessary, get feedback from trusted others.

> **Tip:** For hair washing – Use a screen or shampoo visor to keep water and soap away from face. Meanwhile build tolerance for water in face by deliberately spraying or putting drops of water on your face.
>
> For hair combing – Post a picture showing how you should look if hair is combed satisfactorily. Use the same strategy for dressing.

Use a laminated checklist to ensure that you remember to use soap, shower gel, shampoo, conditioner, as well as possibly dandruff control shampoo, lotions or creams, deodorant, etc.

Sample Hygiene Checklist

Task	Done
Brush teeth for _____ minutes	
Wash face (with soap)	
Shower with soap	
Wash hair (dandruff shampoo?)	
Shave (woman)	
Shave (man)	
Use deodorant	
Use cologne or perfume	
Comb or brush hair	
Have comb or brush with you	
Use makeup?	
Nails clean and neat	

Toothbrushing
Use a toothbrush that has a timer if you are having trouble monitoring this task. Consult your dentist for how-tos and a time frame.

Clothing
Dressing appropriately is often challenging for adolescents/adults with AS. Like so many other aspects of life, learning how to dress, to shop for clothes, to coordinate clothing, etc., can be made easier given some guidelines and strategies.

1. To make shopping more manageable, shop at small specialty stores where there is less merchandise to confuse you and more assistance to help you.

2. Buy coordinates, outfits, sets.

3. Shop online.

4. Have someone pre-select or bring home outfits for you to try on.

5. When shopping, bring along a trusted friend or coach.

6. To ensure that your dress is appropriate:

   - Make sure clothes are clean and pressed.

   - Ask or look at pictures in magazines such as *Newsweek, Time, Seventeen, Glamour*. Notice what others are wearing (at school or at the office; during the day; at the theatre or opera; at a restaurant) to determine what type of attire is appropriate for the situation. For example, for an interview, wear a suit or a nice dress/pant set; for a relaxed barbeque, wear jeans, casual wear.

   - Use coordinates, sets and outfits. Many clothes come together as sets – matching tops and bottoms or coordinating/complementary tops and bottoms. This makes it simple to put together an outfit without wondering if things go together.

   - Make and follow specific rules such as wear only patterned items on top OR bottom (unless a set) with solid color (from pattern) to match.

Clothing Worksheet

Situation or Event	Source of Information	Apparel Selected	Check
Workplace	Observation	Pants outfit	
Wedding	Consult with sister	Evening dress	

Once you have an idea of what kind of clothes you will need, be sure you have all the "components" of the outfit.

Clothing Checklist

Item	Condition – I have item (clean and ironed, not torn) or needs to be obtained/purchased	Check
Dress or pants and top		
Shoes to match		
Socks, stockings, pantyhose, knee highs		
Accessories (jewelry, scarf)		
Purse appropriate for event		
Outerwear (jacket, coat)		
Appropriate undergarments		

Tip: Create a cue card or strategy page for this.

Hair/Grooming

Pick a style that is easy for you to care for and is flattering for your body type and looks. Make sure you keep a comb or brush with you, and always check your hair when you come in from being outdoors or when you take a hat off.

Consult a hairdresser or barber for advice about hair cut/hair care/style.

Laundry

How often to do laundry depends on how many clothes you have – you should always have 2-3 days of clean underwear and clothes available. Change bed linens weekly, towels after two uses – consider putting this on your weekly schedule. Depending on the type of clothes you wear, they may need to be pressed or ironed after being washed. As a general rule, stay away from clothes that require much care unless you can afford to send them to a dry cleaner for proper treatment.

Getting up Independently in the Morning

If this is an area of difficulty, try different methods, including alternatives to alarm clocks such as:

- lamp that is set on a timer to shine a bright light
- progressive clock that wakes you gradually with light, peaceful sounds and aroma (Hammacher Schlemmer – www.hammacherschlemmer.com)
- music rather than alarm
- Clocky – a rolling alarm clock that "jumps" off onto the floor and makes you chase it around to turn it off!

Getting Ready to Live on Your Own

As you anticipate living independently, it is advisable that you move through a sequence of intermediary steps rather than making an abrupt move. You can prepare for living on your own by using resources in your environment to practice in the real world. Let's look at some examples.

- Start by sleeping away from home to get used to it; for example,
  a. Sleep over at a relative or friend's house
  b. House-sit for a relative or friend
  c. Stay alone in your own house
  d. Stay in a hotel for a night
  e. Gradually increase the number of nights you sleep away from home
  f. Rent a room in a friend or relative's house
  g. Take a very short-term lease or rent month-to-month before committing to a one- or two-year lease

- Consider accessibility to supermarkets, drug stores, and transportation if you don't drive (consider parking availability if you have a car)

- Consider proximity to parents or other helping adults

- Consider plans to avoid isolation

- Review the new responsibilities you will have and practice these new tasks and skills:
  - Bill paying
  - Shopping
  - Medical care
  - Transportation
  - Safety
  - Cleaning
  - Laundry
  - Cooking

These are all transition steps to try before making a major move. You want to feel comfortable that you can manage on your own in one of these intermediary situations before you make a more "permanent" arrangement. You also want to know that your plans work (i.e., you can get to the supermarket, you can take care of your bills). This means that you monitor how well things are going and that you "test drive" the situation for a reasonable length of time (for example, 6 months).

This is a time when a supportive adult, coach or mentor can be helpful in delineating steps towards independence and evaluating how well you have mastered the skills you are working on developing.

Transportation

Many AS adolescents/adults have difficulty with spatial orientation, directionality, etc. They may get lost easily or lack awareness of what is going on around them, which puts them at greater risk for accidents, even as pedestrians. It can be particularly challenging when utilizing public transportation systems or driving. However, this too can be tackled by, once again, starting small.

Here is a list of strategies to try out in an effort to improve or compensate for poor spatial orientation/directionality.

- Draw a map or download one from the Internet. Now use visualization techniques; that is, try to picture in your mind going down the streets you will be traversing, getting to intersections, watching and waiting until it is safe to proceed. In this way you are "rehearsing" the route and will feel more familiar with it when you actually set out.

- Practice crossing a busy corridor at school or in a mall or office building before attempting to cross a street.

- Make yourself (or have someone else make) "treasure hunts" using simple maps for you to follow.

- Target a specific destination to get to on your own (with no streets to cross initially, if necessary) (around the corner, down the street) and practice getting there independently. Then try a longer, more challenging route.

- Use verbal mediation to describe your planned route. As for the visualization technique, you "pretend" to follow the route by describing it in words. For example, "I am walking down Main Street passing the post office. I am approaching the corner of Adams Street. I will be turning right on Adams Street …" This method also helps you feel familiar with your route before you even begin.

- Take short trips on a bus or subway first with someone, then on your own, with someone waiting at the destination.

- Practice noticing things in traffic – observe what kinds of things happen and how they are responded to.

- If planning to drive your own car, use an adaptive driving instructor or occupational therapist to help, advise, instruct and monitor your driving.

> **Tip:** When walking anywhere, be the "guide" and announce what is coming up – what dangers might be present, what actions to take. Do this in a variety of situations as a way of getting in the habit of noticing, evaluating, responding.

Implement (Have you mastered the needed skill? Move on or revise the approach, as needed).

Applying Skills You Have Learned:
Combining Vision-Goal-Plan (VGP) with PAPI

Life is constantly changing, and new situations arise all the time. A combination of the two processes discussed – VGP (vision to goal to plan) and PAPI (Predict, Anticipate, Plan and Implement) – can be employed to manage these new situations such as:

- Graduation
- Post-graduate life
- New living arrangements
- Social life
- Leisure activities
- Relationships
- Social events
- Obtaining and maintaining friendships
- Employment
  - Obtaining work
  - Functioning successfully at work
- Interviews
  - College
  - Job

Let's look at an example.

Postsecondary Planning

Predict:
> I might not be ready to go away from home.
> I might find dorm life stressful.
> I need a challenging, intellectual environment.

Anticipate:
What social, organizational and independent life skills will I need?
Evaluate the options for postsecondary education relative to skills that you have already mastered versus those still needed. If college is a potential and desirable next step, you will want to *prepare* by developing the independent life skills and the pre-academic (organizational) and academic skills you will need. You will also need to determine what *accommodations* (such as a single dorm room) you may need the postsecondary program to provide.

If you anticipate that college may not be the best choice for you at this time, consider other options. For example,

- Would you benefit from a post-graduate year?
- How about commuting to a local school or community college?
- Are you ready to take a full load, or would it be better to take a reduced course load?
- What about online or distance (correspondence) learning?
- Would you be interested in an internship? (a paid or unpaid "job" where the focus is on learning and deciding if the job is appropriate for you to pursue)
- How about a transition program? (a program designed to help prepare (academically, organizationally, socially, psychologically) for a next step
- Is there a suitable school or program that could be accessed if you were living with a family friend or relative?
- Would a supported college program be doable?

Parents, educators and clinicians are recognizing that many young people on the spectrum are not ready to go on to college directly from high school and may need a "gap" year and alternative experiences to prepare them to move on. Many new and interesting programs are being developed throughout the country to provide viable alternatives to immediate transition to college. See the Appendix for additional information.

Plan:
After you have gathered information, you will begin to make your **plan** by selecting one of the options you have investigated.

Implement:
Once you have made a plan that seems desirable and feasible, you begin the process of **implementing** your plan (apply to college or program, or whatever fits).

Get advice and counseling about your choices. You can consult school counselors, private or public agencies that provide such services, local groups and organizations concerned with AS, or trusted relatives or friends.

It would also be beneficial to visit a variety of programs in order to assess how appropriate they might be for you. Start by visiting and studying websites. Call or email to arrange a visit. Ask for "references;" that is, people who have recently completed the program or are currently enrolled. Develop questions about what you want to know. Arrange for an interview with these folks if possible.

Social Life, Relationships and Friendships

This can be a tough one. You want some friends, significant others – a social life. How do you start?

Levels of Relationships

First, acquaint yourself with the levels of relationships. You can think of it as an upside-down triangle.

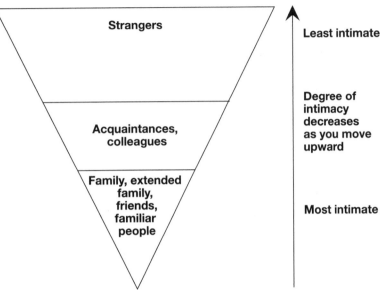

You can also think of it as concentric circles in which the smallest group is at the center.

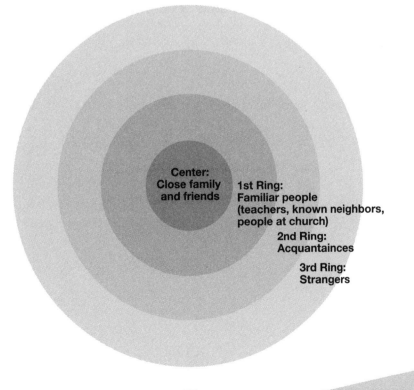

"Rules" of Behavior for Each Level

The degree of intimacy you can display and allow another to exhibit toward you increases as you move down the triangle or inward from the outer rim of the circles. The smallest number of people are close family and friends: parents, siblings, grandparents, special relatives and close friends of long standing. With these people, you can be maximally open; you can tell them private thoughts and feelings. You can hug them and show affection openly.

Relationships with persons from the second level of extended family and friends, familiar people (colleagues, church members, neighbors), require you to be a bit more cautious about what you reveal about yourself, your life and your family. You might greet them with a hug or a handshake, but it would be briefer and less intense.

The rules for relating to people on the third level of acquaintances require you to be pleasant and polite, yet reserved in your interactions. Very limited physical contact (handshake) is appropriate. Conversations tend to be light and shallow – small talk and general information.

With strangers, behavior depends on the setting in which they are encountered. If you meet at work, through friends, at a party or event, you might consider them impending acquaintances. A friendly, yet careful approach without physical contact would be acceptable. If it is someone on the street, in a coffee shop or other public place, it is probably preferable to remain aloof and restrict interaction to a nod or to refrain from responding at all.

Who is in your world? Fill in the names of people in each category using the triangle model below or the circle model on page 75.

What Are Your Relationships?

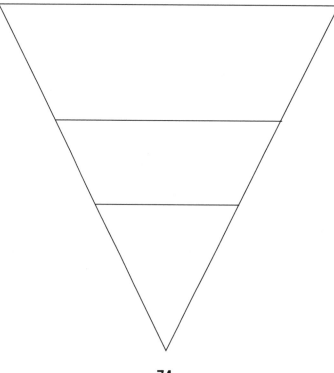

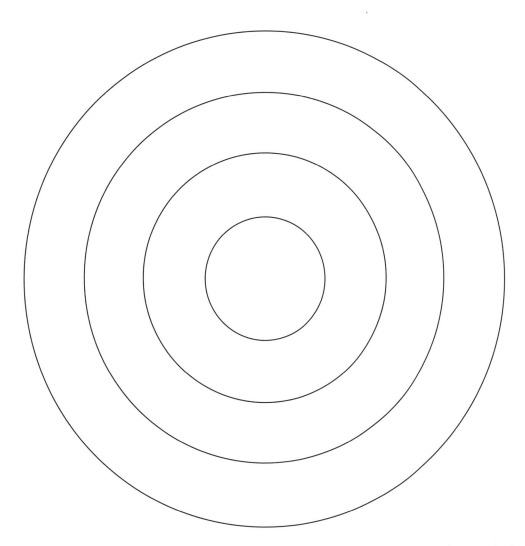

Now take a look at your diagram and evaluate the information you have written relative to your hopes and dreams – your goals – as they relate to social relationships.

- Are there any friends in the center of the circle or at the tip of the triangle? _____

- Would you like someone to be there? _____

- Do you have some acquaintances? _____

- Do you have enough acquaintances, or do you want to feel closer to someone? Is there someone in the acquaintance group who has the potential to move into the more intimate category?

Can you tell what distinguishes an acquaintance from a friend? Do you know the "rules" for each level of a relationship and what behaviors would be associated with each level? Do you know how people move further in or out of the circle?

These are questions for which you will need to get answers in order to begin the process of developing and deepening relationships.

Rules for Levels of Relationships

There are different rules for the different groups of people. Can you explain some of the rules you know about how to interact with people? For example,

Close family and friends:

_____

_____

_____

Familiar people (clergy, family friends, teachers, etc.):

_____

_____

_____

Coworkers:

_____

_____

_____

Acquaintances:

_____

_____

_____

Strangers:

_____

_____

_____

Conversational "Small Talk"

In order to be able to contribute to conversations, you must have some "common knowledge." To identify some topics, try a Venn diagram (A Venn diagram consists of two or more overlapping circles that show a group of items/people that share common characteristics; it is intended to help you organize and systematize. It originated in mathematics "set theory.")

List some of your interests in the left circle – be specific. For example, don't just write "music." Name the specific type of music. The same goes for books, movies, etc. Then, based on questioning or observing neurotypical age-mates, list some of their interests in the right-hand circle. An example is given below.

Sample

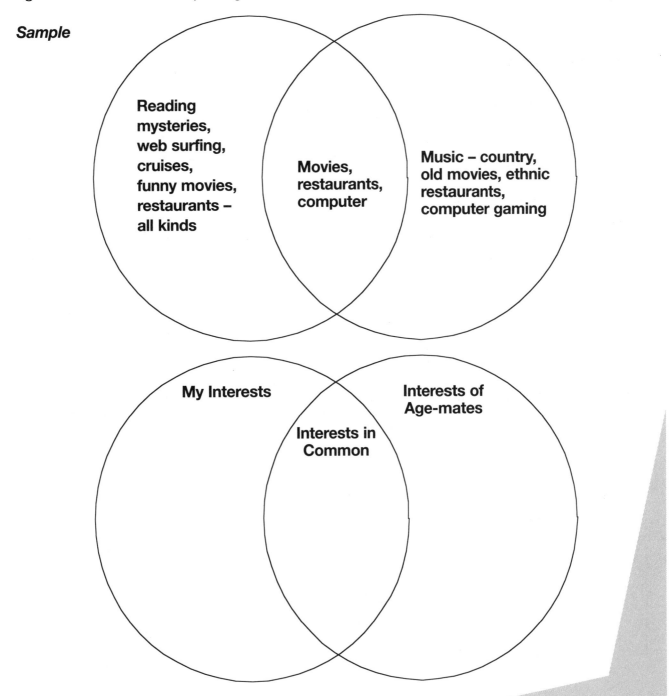

Tip: People with AS frequently reveal that they don't know what to say in conversations and that they don't know much about the topics being discussed. Many people with AS have narrow special interests but lack broader knowledge of the everyday world around them.

It is helpful to expand your knowledge of the world around you and to broaden your knowledge base. In this way, you are more likely to have something to say and to be able to participate in general conversations. An excellent source of "common knowledge" is the *Dictionary of Cultural Literacy* (Houghton Mifflin, 1993). This, and similar volumes, will give you lots of good information people presume you know and will enable you to comment on a broad range of topics.

It is important that conversations be reciprocal; that is, you must listen to what the other person(s) is/are saying, and your response must be connected. You must avoid "making speeches" about your special interests, but instead engage in a discourse about a subject of mutual interest. For example, if you find somebody who likes movies, listen to what she talks about before you launch into your own special interest about old camera techniques, if, in fact, the other person is more interested in the plot or story line and how it relates to her own life.

Monitoring What You Say

Another caution is that you must screen some of what you say. Not everything that comes to your mind should come out of your mouth. *Think before you speak.* Ask for a minute to give you time to formulate your response.

The following template may help.

Appropriate Responses – Leftover Feelings

Situation	What I want to say	What I can say	What to do with leftover feelings (how can you express yourself appropriately or get your feelings out?)

Relationships – Going to the Next Level

How can you tell whether you like or are liked by someone? Many people with AS have trouble recognizing feelings, both their own and the feelings of others. One way to tell if there is potential in a relationship is to assess how much work it is to be with and to interact with another person. Because it is often such hard work to be with others, a good sign of a promising relationship is the degree of comfort you experience. In other words, the more comfortable you feel with someone, the greater the potential that you can have a satisfying relationship with him or her.

Comfort level suggests that you feel "in sync" with the other person, that you are accepted by the other person and that you are accepting of him or her.

If you are interested in being friends with someone, you must move from "small talk" into more personal conversation – you must shift from "what " questions (what happened? what did you do?) to "why," "how," "what did you think" questions (how did you feel about …?, what do you think of …?). Also, you must be prepared to talk about your thoughts and feelings (I thought …, I felt …).

It's up to you to decide what you want your social life to be. Some people want more contact with other people; enjoy interactions more; need more stimulation. There's no right or wrong here. Consider the following.

How Many Relationships Do You Want?
How Close Do You Want to Get with Others?

From the following, select which type of relationship you wish to have.

1. I want to get out of the house and be around people.

2. I want to participate in an enjoyable activity with other people.

3. I want to meet people who share my interests.

4. I want to have someone to go to the movies with.

5. I want to feel close to someone.

6. I want to love and be loved.

7. I want a sexual partner.

Once you know what you want (once you have set your social goal), you can begin to work on achieving it. Considering the selection you made above, how would you characterize your social goal(s)?

_____

_____

_____

_____

_____

To create your plan, consider what actions you might take to achieve your goal(s).

Which of the following would help you achieve the above goals (some may apply to more than one goal):

- Work on sensory issues, particularly tactile defensiveness
- Take an adult education class
- Join a group or club that meets regularly
- Ask one member of a group, class or club to have coffee, go for a drink, etc.
- Go to a movie, a lecture, a concert or a museum
- Learn to recognize how you feel when with _____. Try to experience the feeling associated with feeling words
- Figure out who you are interested (really interested) in knowing more about and who you feel most comfortable with

Developing relationships begins with determining where the relationship is at the beginning (where on the triangle or in the circles) and working from there toward the middle. Let's say, for example, that you join the Science Fiction Club. In the club you meet one or two people who seem "nice." You invite one or the other (or both) to go for coffee after the meeting – or to meet for a meal before the meeting. You go through the preliminary "small talk," and if everybody agrees to meet again like that, in subsequent "dates" you start deepening the conversations with relatively simple "I" statements: "I like New York in June, how about you?" and by asking feeling questions such as "what was it like to _____?" or "how does it feel to _____"?

> **Tip:** Small talk is tough because it often seems meaningless and perfunctory. You can make it meaningful by asking yourself what you would like to know about the other person and what you think he or she would like to know about you. Then ask questions based on genuine interest rather than perfunctory, "standard" questions.

Dating

The transition from friendship to dating is sometimes so subtle that many people with AS don't notice the change. In fact, some people on the spectrum ask, "How do I know when things have changed?"

Very often, dating involves touching of one kind or another. For example, holding hands, patting on the shoulder, putting arms around each other, hugging and kissing are common ways for people to express their affection for each other. For somebody with AS, the timetable for physical expressions may be considerably delayed and may require work on sensory issues (such as tactile defensiveness) in order for them to be able to tolerate the physical closeness.

Going to the next level in a relationship involves the same process (VGP) we have discussed throughout this workbook: vision, goals, evaluation, plan.

What is your vision/goal: Do you want to be dating? Evaluate: What skills do you need? What gets in the way? Of particular importance when considering moving into a physical relationship is safety (health concerns such as AIDS and STDs) as well as the sincerity of your potential partner (does this person genuinely care about you, or is he or she taking advantage of you for financial or sexual gain?). How long have you known each other? How consistent has the other person's concern and support been? (Does the person respond supportively when you are ill or feeling sad? Does he ask how things are going, wait for your answer, respond to your response?) How respectful is the person of your feelings? (Does she ask your opinion, ask how you feel about things, apologize if she inadvertently hurt your feelings?) How much do you know about the person? What kind of information do you have? Have you met family members? How intimate are you prepared to be? Do you agree on the pace of the physical relationship?

These are important questions to address before embarking on a physical relationship. If you are not sure what to do, this is a good time to consult some of the allies you have identified earlier.

Once you've made the decision to deepen the relationship, you can develop your plan. This will require collaboration between you and your significant other; you will need to talk about it and come to some agreement that you both want the same things and that you "are on the same page" relative to a timetable. You may want to consult your family or a professional who knows you; you may want to go to a counselor together to talk about how to proceed.

Relationships – Love

Many people on the spectrum struggle to discern degrees of feelings, including love. They find it an elusive concept. One woman I knew had several children, but had never told them she loved them because she didn't know what love felt like and she didn't want to lie to them. Learning to recognize love is difficult but doable.

If you've followed the process of making friends, deepening the relationship and dating presented above, you may be at a point of wondering whether you love or are in love with someone.

First of all, it is important to think about the differences between fantasy and real life. Because of the black-and-white thinking that is typical of people with AS, some Aspies find it difficult to recognize loving and caring feelings. They report that the "signal is too weak." They expect to be "swept away," to be overcome with romantic euphoria. In the absence of such an unlikely fairy-tale scenario, they may overlook growing feelings of love. Don't fall prey to this misapprehension.

So, what does it feel like to deeply care about, to love someone?

For people on the spectrum who have trouble recognizing feelings, there are somewhat different indices. Here are some ways to begin to tell.

Being with people is often described by Aspies as "hard work" (stressful and contrived, unnatural and exhausting). But being with certain people is "easier," more comfortable, less stressful, not as hard work. There is less anxiety and agitation. Such feelings of enjoyment and comfort may be indicators of caring and loving feelings, and could be the beginning of a closer relationship.

Learning to recognize and distinguish between some of these feelings (how I feel when I am with certain people) may help you acquire a better understanding of words like "love." It is important to remember that your experience of "love" may be very different from others', but nonetheless equally genuine.

Spend a little time reflecting on what you feel when you are with

- Parent(s)

- Sibling(s)

- Close relatives

- Favorite teachers, mentor or coach?

- Friends

Try to be specific in the words you choose to describe your feelings: calm, comforted, etc. Ask others to help you come up with ideas (you can use a thesaurus to help you find words that might fit). Then you might practice learning how to recognize these feelings by prompting yourself to "name" the feeling you are experiencing at various times.

When I am with someone I think I care about/like/love, I feel:

_____

_____

_____

Of course, there are different kinds of love: love of parents, siblings, romantic love. Stephen Shore's books, *Ask and Tell* and *Beyond the Wall,* as well as Zosia Zaks's *Life and Love: Positive Strategies for Autistic Adults* (www.asperger.net) are excellent resources for information on relationships on the autism spectrum.

> **Tip:** Even for neurotypicals, dating and romantic relationships can be challenging, due to the many nuances of feelings and emotions. Above all, never push yourself on somebody (stalking is, in fact, illegal) if he or she makes it clear that your advances are not welcome.

Work – Getting and Keeping It

Obtaining and maintaining meaningful and appropriate employment can be extremely challenging for people on the spectrum. Some statistics (National Autistic Society of Great Britain; http://www.autism.org.uk/) suggest that only 6% of people with an autism spectrum disorder have full-time paid employment. Of this number, we can assume that many are "underemployed;" that is, engaged in work that is not commensurate with their ability. This is a pretty appalling situation.

What accounts for this?

There are many factors. Some folks with AS have difficulty figuring out a good "match" and try to do jobs for which they are ill suited or ill prepared. Some people have great difficulty with interviews and, therefore, never even get the opportunity to demonstrate their abilities. Others get hired but have a tendency to misunderstand, make mistakes or have problems interacting with bosses and coworkers and, therefore, don't keep their jobs.

The process of identifying what has interfered with your ability to get and keep work will enable you to manage this aspect of your life better. Again, the combination of VGP (Vision-Goal-Plan) and PAPI (Predict, Anticipate, Prepare, Implement) can guide you through the process of finding, obtaining and keeping employment.

Let's look at how this works.

Getting a Job

Start with a vision; what kind of work do you see yourself doing? To develop your vision, use information from the profile you have constructed in this workbook with a special emphasis on

1. tasks that you find enjoyable
2. the setting you are most comfortable with
3. the degree of interaction required vs. what you are comfortable with
4. a realistic assessment of your strengths and preferences

You have generated some of this information earlier in this workbook – refer to the section What Do I Really Like to Do and in What Contexts?

Utilizing this information and keeping an open mind, consider jobs that might match your profile. The *Occupational Outlook Handbook* (www.bls.gov/oco/) can be useful in identifying jobs you might not be aware of.

Record some of your thoughts and ideas here.

I love to: _____
Example: work on the computer, solve puzzles

I am most comfortable: _____
Example: in a small office with people I know well

I prefer: _____
Example: to work alone or with one other person

I am good at: _____

A job that might fit this profile could be:_____

If you need help with this aspect of your planning, consult some of the many vocational guidance services, both agencies and individuals, that can provide occupational assessments, guidance, coaching and job placement. Look online or in the telephone book under Social Service or Vocational Guidance.

If you now have a **vision** of appropriate employment and your **goal** is to obtain it, your **plan** should be twofold:

1. Work on the skills you will need (interview skills, tolerance for some group work) in that particular job, and
2. Work on obtaining the job itself.

Step 1: Use PAPI to analyze the job and to prepare for the interview.

> **Predict** what is likely to be asked of you in the performance of the job.
> **Anticipate** problems you might encounter.
> **Prepare** yourself for performing the tasks you have identified.
> **Implement** your plan.

Step 2: Prepare a resumé and cover letter. Use models you find online or in books to guide you (see Appendix). Make sure someone else critiques and proofreads it.

Step 3: Consult an employment agency or employment advertisements in your local newspaper or online (craigslist.org, monster.com) to locate potential positions. Asking friends and acquaintances is also a good idea at this stage.

Step 4: Send a letter and resumé to job offerings that appeal to you. Follow up with an email or a phone call.

Step 5: If you obtain an interview, prepare for the interview, including writing down some questions you can ask to demonstrate that you have true interest and have done some research into the company/place of employment.

Step 6: On the day of the interview ...

- Dress appropriately for the interview.
- Bring extra resumés and have something in your hands (pen and pad) to avoid "fiddling" of fidgeting.
- Greet the interviewer with direct eye contact, a firm handshake and a semblance of a smile.
- Make sure you understand what will be expected of you as the job is described to you. Ask questions to obtain specificity and clarification. Write things down. Be prepared with questions that indicate you have done some research about the company or position.
- Acknowledge obvious problems – if you yawn when you're nervous and start yawning, say so (e.g., "Sometimes I yawn when I'm nervous; I hope you can overlook that")
- Refer to your resumé to deflect from any weaknesses in the way you are presenting yourself. Consider saying something like "I don't always come across so well in an interview, but as you can see from my resumé ..."

Step 7: Write a thank-you note on business stationery for the interview. Follow up in a week with a phone call regarding the status of your application.

Keeping a Job

Once you have been hired, you will need to ...

- clarify expectations, such as asking for specific directions and guidelines about hours, responsibilities, workplace rules, procedures
- write things down – tasks, procedures, rules – and post them near your work space
- ask for clarification and feedback as you proceed or upon completion of a task (" I hope that was what you were looking for; " "Let me know if you'd like any changes").
- familiarize yourself and strictly adhere to the unspoken rules and culture of the workplace (consult *The Hidden Curriculum* by Brenda Smith Myles, Melissa Trautman, and Ronda Schelvan (www.asperger.net). For example,
  - Arrive on time
  - Take only permissible breaks
  - Dress appropriately (see section on dressing and hygiene); make sure you are neat and clean and that your clothes reflect attention to the weather and the setting
  - Be cordial and polite
  - Keep your work space organized and neat

> **Tip:** It is a good idea to have work done in advance of the deadline. In this way you would be able to show the work to the supervisor and make any adjustments that may be needed in time for the deadline. It also helps in case something unexpected happens.

- when given instructions, rephrase to make sure you understand ("So what I need to do is …")
- schedule tasks – ask coworkers to help you set the amount of time needed for tasks if you are unsure
- build in checkpoints to ensure that you will meet deadlines
- build in breaks and interaction-free time to forestall overload. Don't wait until it's too late; it's not when you feel you need the break that you need it – be proactive – if you take breaks before you actually need them, you won't need them!

> **Tip:** If you reach a breaking point, have and use a plan (i.e., your emergency kit, your "safe haven"). DO NOT melt down in public. You can do this!

On the Road to Success

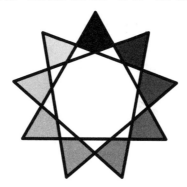

You've done a lot of thinking and writing by now. To be successful you must:

- be motivated to "get a life"
- be able to identify (observe) "normative" (neurotypical) behavior and to evaluate your own behavior in relation to it
- be willing to try the "un-natural" – try out new approaches and strategies, albeit unfamiliar, potentially uncomfortable, and contrived

No matter how well you have planned, there might still be some obstacles to overcome. This next section introduces some of the stumbling blocks you might encounter and ways to cope with them.

Roadblocks to Change

There are several potential roadblocks to change inherent in the AS profile. Of particular note is the fear that changes in behavior will compromise your identity. Despite loneliness and disappointment with social and everyday functioning, most people with AS become accustomed to their "quirky" image. In many cases, they are proud of their differences, even though they may also be frustrated and saddened by the consequences of their differences. They are fearful of losing the "self they know."

Evading Roadblocks

Distinguishing between your "core identity" (the components of your essential self) and the "satellite" characteristics that can be manipulated/modified without eroding your core identity can be sufficiently reassuring to enable you to make some adjustments in behavior. By "core identity" we are talking about the inner qualities that define you as a person such as intelligence, kindness, love of animals and nature, versus external qualities such as hairstyle, clothes, fear of flying, which can be changed without changing the essence of the person.

You can change many things and still be yourself. You can change your physical appearance, interests, likes and dislikes, activities and behaviors and still be you. You define who you are and what components define you.

Your Core Identity

A way to conceptualize this is to look at the Core Identity Model below. Here you create a visual of what you (and others) believe are the components of the "essential you" versus the characteristics and behaviors that can be modified without eroding your identity.

Core Identity Model

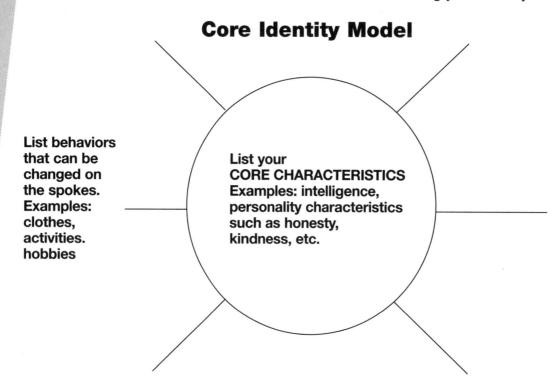

List behaviors that can be changed on the spokes. Examples: clothes, activities. hobbies

List your CORE CHARACTERISTICS Examples: intelligence, personality characteristics such as honesty, kindness, etc.

In the blank form below, first list your core characteristics in the circle. Then on the spokes, list behaviors that can be changed without compromising your core identity.

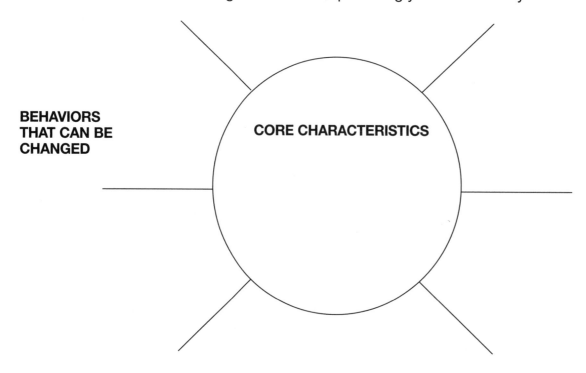

BEHAVIORS THAT CAN BE CHANGED

CORE CHARACTERISTICS

Ask a trusted friend, therapist, coach or relative to comment on your choices. Then go back and consider the list of things that you feel can be changed.

Examine your diagram. Have some of the behaviors that can be changed been problematic (e.g., style of dress – you always wear sweatpants because they are comfortable, but they have been inappropriate in several circumstances such as job interviews). For each of these problematic but changeable behaviors, consider an alternative that might be more successful but that will not change your core identity.

List of problematic but changeable behaviors:

1. _____

2. _____

3. _____

4. _____

5. _____

Devise a plan to modify these behaviors in order to achieve your goal(s) while preserving your core identity.

More Roadblocks

Despite genuine motivation to improve their quality of life, some characteristics of individuals with AS operate as constraints. Let's look at some of them.

RIGIDITY – Many individuals with AS get "stuck" or hyper-focused on a belief, idea or activity. They tend to think concretely in black-and-white terms, unable to see options or "gray areas." They may become perseverative, returning to the same stance or idea over and over.

To effect change, you must recognize (acknowledge) these tendencies and seek ways to avert/forestall them.

Do you recognize this tendency in yourself? _____

Can you give some examples?

_____

_____

Things are not always "black" or "white." There are steps or options in between. For example, you want to see a movie, but your friend wants to go out for dinner. What are the intermediary options?

_____

_____

What can you try to do when you sense that you are being inflexible?

_____

_____

In addition to what you have come up with yourself, consider the following suggestions:

1. Create a visual of the possibilities – ask for help if you can't perceive them.

Black	Gradations & Options	White

Practice the skill of "filling in the blanks" in a variety of situations. Make it a game – how many options can you identify in Situation X?

2. Learn to shift gears: tolerate ambiguity and interruptions by practicing some of the following:

- Listen to TV and radio simultaneously and shift back and forth in order to follow the "story;"
- Listen to a story and do math problems (or any two activities) – again, shifting attention to sustain connections to both;
- Set up planned interruptions at agreed-upon times. Later set up unexpected interruptions you have agreed to tolerate; ask your trusted ally to randomly interrupt you with the agreement that you both understand that initially this may be very difficult and that you will try not to "melt down," get upset or blame them.
- Use the call waiting function on the phone to help you shift gears. Arrange for someone to call you during another phone call. Do this several times as a way of learning how to handle interruptions, multitask, set priorities (should I answer the second call and put the first on hold? Should I finish my initial conversation and let the second caller leave a message?).

Have you tried any of these? _____

What helps? _____

What else can you try? _____

_____

Other potential roadblocks to tackle include:

- fearfulness – difficulty with change
- anxiety – strong preference for the familiar
- few resources – limited income, narrow exposure to the world, mainstream culture, life options
- few people to offer help and support

Who can help you? _____

_____

Another Note About Parents

To enhance the collaboration between you and your parents, it is helpful to have both a Plan A and a Plan B for your next steps and to work with your parents and other significant adults to help them understand that you DO have a plan, what steps you are taking, what your time frame is, what alternatives you have in mind, etc.

Use this template to illustrate your Plan A, along with your timetable and corresponding steps to take. Also include an alternative (Plan B).

Making a Plan

Plan A	Timeline and Steps	Alternative (Plan B)
To obtain job as librarian in public library	Apply for jobs listed on Craigslist.com & Monster.com, *The New York Times* & *The Boston Globe.* If no success by December 2007, switch to Plan B.	Apply to a graduate school program to be qualified to be a librarian in a school setting. In preparation for Plan B, take the GRE and obtain information about graduate programs.

Disclosure: To Do or Not to Do

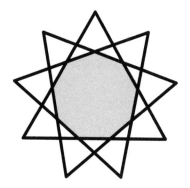

A final consideration in the process of obtaining employment and, generally, improving the quality of your life is the question of disclosure. Under what circumstances, if any, is it advisable to reveal that you have been diagnosed with an autism spectrum disorder?

Each person diagnosed with an autism spectrum disorder faces this question over and over throughout his/her life. How you respond is a complex and very personal decision. Aspies such a Stephen Shore and Zosia Zaks (www.asperger.net) have written extensively on this subject. Refer to their works for more detailed information.

For our purposes here, it is important to explore:

- when it might be appropriate to consider disclosure
- under what circumstances you might disclose
- to whom you might feel it is necessary to disclose
- how to go about disclosing

Think about the people in your world, those listed on the triangle or concentric circles on pages 74 and 75. This is important because the need for disclosure and the way you might go about disclosing to others differ according to where people fall on these models; that is, how close they are to you, what role they play in your life and the nature of the relationship.

Let's illustrate with some examples.

Disclosure

Your close family and friends probably already know that you have AS. What did/do you tell them?

_____

_____

_____

_____

Ask them to describe how they would define AS or how they would explain what they see in you.

_____

_____

_____

_____

_____

Now figure out under what set of circumstances you feel it would be necessary, or you think it would be a good idea, to tell people about AS. What situations can you think of?

1. _____

2. _____

3. _____

4. _____

5. _____

What would you do in each of these situations?

1. _____

2. _____

3. _____

4. _____

5. _____

Each person has to decide for him or herself if, when, and how to disclose. It is my bias that it is pretty hard to "hide" AS. People will notice things and make judgments and, sadly, these judgments are usually incorrect. Disclosure is a way of "putting the cards on the table." This is who I am. I have many strengths and some weaknesses, and here's what they are. Although there are risks involved, especially in the workplace, there are many benefits, including protections under the American Disabilities Act. Consult www.eeoc.gov/facts/fs-ada.html for information.

How best to decide:

- Read about this issue on the websites and in the books mentioned in this text as well as those listed on the web sites listed in the Resources section at the end of the book.

- Talk to other Aspies and people affiliated with your local AS organizations.

- Consult a disability attorney or disability advocate or agency in your area.

- Discuss with close family and friends.

This is a very important decision. So don't be hasty – get good advice. Consider all points of view – try to have an open mind.

If you have made the decision to disclose, here are some possible ways to do so:

General Disclosure Statement
(Oral or written)

You may have noticed _____. I have a type of learning disability (or social disability) (called Asperger Syndrome) that makes _____ difficult. It will help if (you) (I) _____ (take my time) (give me a minute to think) etc.

I'm sorry I _____. It is part of my "social dyslexia" (called AS). I hope you will let me know when _____.

I know that I _____. Sometimes I need_____ to help me _____. It's due to my AS.

Tip: Put the statement on a cue card or in a notebook.

What would you feel comfortable saying?

To employers:

_____

_____

_____

_____

To coworkers:

_____

_____

_____

_____

To acquaintances or neighbors:

_____

_____

_____

_____

Others: (List who they are)

_____

_____

_____

_____

Here are some samples of written statements that may be used if you decide to give more information to people at work or in other parts of your life.

The first is designed to disclose your diagnosis; the second, which is similar, is intended to give additional information without specifically disclosing the diagnosis.

Disclosure Statement Revealing Diagnosis

To:_____

From: _____

Date: _____

In order to promote the most productive working environment, I would like to share some information with you.

I have been diagnosed with _____.

This manifests itself in _____

_____

In the workplace, it is helpful for me to

_____

_____

Some things that may interfere with optimal performance are:

_____

_____

I am capable, qualified and committed to doing the best job possible. It would be helpful to receive feedback and guidance to be sure that I am meeting expectations. (I am working with a coach on issues that may develop.)

Please feel free to discuss this information with me.

Disclosure Statement Without Revealing Diagnosis

To:_____

From: _____

Date: _____

In order to promote the most productive working environment, I would like to share some information with you. I have found that there are things that enhance my performance while other factors may hinder my efforts.

In the workplace, it is helpful for me to: _____

_____

Some things that may interfere with optimal performance are: _____

_____

_____

I am capable, qualified and committed to doing the best job possible. It would be helpful to receive feedback and guidance to ensure that I am meeting expectations. (I am working with a coach on issues that may develop.)

Please feel free to discuss this information with me.

These are just samples; you may want to draft your own statement. Take a stab at it right here.

_____

_____

_____

_____

_____

_____

_____

_____

_____

_____

_____

_____

Final Thoughts

This workbook was intended to aid you in a journey of self-discovery. It is my hope that you have found it useful in learning about yourself and that it has given you some ideas about how to achieve the quality of life you are entitled to and that you desire.

I would enjoy hearing from you if you have comments or suggestions. You can write me in care of the Autism Asperger Publishing Company, P.O. Box 23173, Shawnee Mission, KS 66283.

I believe that most of what does not come intuitively can be learned. I hope that you are having success as you make your journey.

Now that you've reached this point in your journey of self-awareness, congratulate yourself and celebrate. To do so, write the letters of your full name vertically along the left margin of the paper below and use adjectives beginning with each letter to describe yourself. I've given you a sample using my name:

Education advocate
Loves chocolate, reading and visiting New York
Lifelong learner
Enjoys traveling and cruises
Needs downtime

Has respect for differences

Keeps too much "stuff"
Obeys the rules
Remembers and loves history
Is committed to helping others
Not a loner but likes being alone

Write one about yourself:

(Please add or delete lines as necessary to fit your name)

Appendix

Supplementary Information
- Postsecondary Options

Templates
- PAPI Protocol
- Goal-Setting
- Task Lists
- Decision-Making Model
- Clothing Worksheet
- Interview Worksheet
- Sample Resumé
- Sample Cover Letter
- Organizers for Managing Tasks of Daily Living
- Telephone
- Travel
- Doctor's Appointments
- Bill Paying
- Independent Life Skills Assessments
- Resources Related to Asperger Syndrome and Autism Spectrum Disorders in General

Supplementary Information

Postsecondary Options

Many teens and young adults on the spectrum feel that they are not ready to go away to a four-year college directly after high school. The following list suggests other options that you may want to consider.

- Commute to local college

- Attend community college and live at home

- Attend transition programs – a program combining supervised independent living, group experiences, internships and college credit

- Attend colleges with support – most colleges and universities provide some form of disability services and counseling

- Enroll in vocational post-graduate programs at local vocational school

- Find full- or part-time employment

- Participate in specialized independent living/college programs – these programs combine supervised living and instruction in life skills with attendance at a nearby community or four-year college or university. Examples include:

  - Brevard Center in Melbourne, Florida (www.brevardcenter.org) or the Berkshire Center in Massachusetts (www.berkshirecenter.org)
  - College Living Experience – now has three locations (Boca Raton, FL; Denver, CO; and Austin, TX) (www.cleinc.net)
  - New York Institute of Technology (www.nyit) Introduction to Independence – Summer Vocational Independence Program
  - Chapel Haven, Connecticut (www.chapelhaven.org) Asperger's Syndrome Adult Transition Program
  - Gersh College Experience – Buffalo, New York (www.gershacademy.org)
  - Eastern New Mexico University Occupational Training Program, Roswell, New Mexico (www.valparint.com)
  - Allen Institute Center for Innovative Learning, Hebron, CT (www.thealleninstitute.org)

- Participate in college internship program – Bloomington Indiana (www.bloomingtoncenter.net)

Templates

PAPI Protocol Template

You have permission to copy this template so you can complete it for various parts of your life.

Predict: (*What new skills will be needed?*)

_____

_____

_____

_____

Anticipate: (*What are the specific differences you will encounter?*)

_____

_____

_____

_____

Prepare: (*Steps must you take to get ready*)

_____

_____

_____

_____

Implement: (*Do it*)

_____

_____

_____

_____

From E. S. Korin (2007). *Asperger Syndrome – An Owner's Manual 2.* Shawnee Mission, KS: Autism Asperger Publishing Company; www.asperger.net. Used with permission.

Goal-Setting Template

(refer to Inspiration software at www.inspiration.com for additional templates)

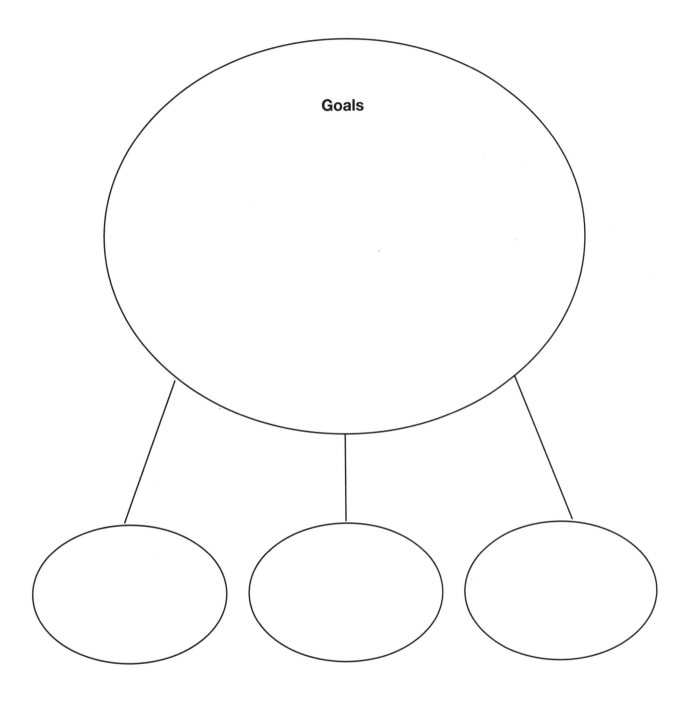

Goals

Task Lists to Laminate

Sample

Task
Brush teeth for _____minutes
Wash face (with soap)
Shower with soap
Wash hair
(dandruff shampoo?)
Shave (woman)
Shave (man)
Use deodorant
Use cologne or perfume
Comb or brush hair
Have comb or brush with you
Use makeup?
Use makeup?
Nails clean and neat

Create Your Own

Task

From E. S. Korin (2007). *Asperger Syndrome – An Owner's Manual 2.* Shawnee Mission, KS: Autism Asperger Publishing Company; www.asperger.net. Used with permission.

Decision-Making Model

Sample

Situation	Rules – written and unwritten	Observations	Protocol
Wedding	Don't wear white		Respond by due date; buy or send present; dress appropriately
Best man at wedding	Give a toast		Write out what you will say
Services in church or synagogue	Wear a head covering? Wear dress clothes (no pants for women)		Be sure to wear appropriate clothing

Create Your Own

Situation	Rules – written and unwritten	Observations	Protocol

From E. S. Korin (2007). *Asperger Syndrome – An Owner's Manual 2.* Shawnee Mission, KS: Autism Asperger Publishing Company; www.asperger.net. Used with permission.

Clothing Worksheet

Sample

Situation or Event	Source of Information	Apparel Selected
Workplace	Observation	Pants outfit
Wedding	Consult with sister	Evening dress

Create Your Own

Situation or Event	Source of Information	Apparel Selected

From E. S. Korin (2007). *Asperger Syndrome – An Owner's Manual 2.* Shawnee Mission, KS: Autism Asperger Publishing Company; www.asperger.net. Used with permission.

Clothing Worksheet (cont.)

Once you have an idea of what kind of clothes you will need, be sure you have all the components of the outfit:

Sample

Item	Condition (You have the item and it is clean and wearable or (You need to purchase the item)	Check
Dress or pants and top		
Shoes to match		
Socks, stockings, pantyhose, knee highs		
Accessories (jewelry, scarf)		
Purse appropriate for event		
Outerwear (jacket, coat)		
Appropriate undergarments (slip, camisole)		

Create Your Own

Item	Condition (clean, mended) or needs to be bought	Check

From E. S. Korin (2007). *Asperger Syndrome – An Owner's Manual 2.* Shawnee Mission, KS: Autism Asperger Publishing Company; www.asperger.net. Used with permission.

Interview Worksheet – College or Job

Predictions of questions:	1.
	2.
	3.
	4.
	5.
Possible Responses:	1.
	2.
	3.
	4.
	5.
Questions I might ask:	1.
	2.
	3.

Ready for an interview?	Check
I am dressed appropriately	
I have needed materials (resumé, paper to write on, pen)	
I know where I am going and know how to get there	
I have combed my hair and I am clean and neat	
I have prepared for this interview by developing some questions	
Other	

From E. S. Korin (2007). *Asperger Syndrome – An Owner's Manual 2.* Shawnee Mission, KS: Autism Asperger Publishing Company; www.asperger.net. Used with permission.

Sample Resumé

Common Elements of Resumé

PERSONAL INFORMATION

NAME
ADDRESS
PHONE   EMAIL
FAX
WEBSITE

BRIEF STATEMENT OF OBJECTIVE:

EDUCATIONAL BACKGROUND

DATES   SCHOOL NAME   DEGREE OR DIPLOMA

EMPLOYMENT HISTORY

DATES   COMPANY   BRIEF DESCRIPTION OF RESPONSIBILITIES

REFERENCES

From E. S. Korin (2007). *Asperger Syndrome – An Owner's Manual 2.* Shawnee Mission, KS: Autism Asperger Publishing Company; www.asperger.net. Used with permission.

Sample Cover Letter

It is best to send a cover letter with your resumé. In your cover letter, you introduce yourself, tell what position you are interested in and give information about yourself that will entice the reader to read your resumé.

Examples of resumés and cover letters may be found on the Internet and in many books.

Refer to www.monster.com as one source of information and free samples or templates for resumes and cover letters. Or search for "resumés" and "cover letters" using Google or some other search engine.

If you are looking for a book, search for resumé writing on www.amazon.com, www.borders.com or www.bn.com.

Organizers for Managing Tasks of Daily Living

I'm a list maker – I just love lists. I have found that writing things down, although not generally the method of choice for people on the spectrum, can be a wonderful way to keep track of information and ease the task at hand. To this end I am including some sample lists and checklists as well as information on websites where these materials can be obtained. These types of checklists are invaluable. You can find many helpful checklists and worksheets online at sites such as www.momcentral.com or www.organizetips.com

You can write your own shopping list using online checklists to guide you, or you can print an online checklist and check off what you need.

Tip: If you create your own checklist, make it match the order of products as they are displayed in your supermarket. For example, if the first aisle is butter, eggs, dairy products, etc., list these items first on your checklist. Do the same for each aisle. An annotated diagram of the supermarket may also help.

For example in my supermarket the first aisle is dairy products, juices and processed meats; the next aisle is salad dressings, tuna, olives and pickles, and so on. As I make the list, I visualize the aisles and write things down in the order I will come to them as I travel through the store.

So, my list might start out like this
> Butter
> Eggs
> Cream cheese
> Cheddar
> Yogurt
> Milk
> Juice
> Etc. …

Use this space to make a sketch of your supermarket

Consult www.organizetips.com for wonderful lists for organizing many areas of your life including a printable grocery shopping list.

Telephone

A common area of challenge for people on the spectrum is use of the telephone. The following list may make it easier to handle phone tasks.

Making Calls

1. Prepare yourself by eliminating or minimizing potential distractions or interrupters in the environment.
2. Have pencil and paper available, along with any papers or bills or other information you may need for this call.
3. Be clear about what you hope to accomplish as a result of the call.
4. Be prepared with opening and closing lines:
   a. Opening
      i. "Hello , this is _____. I am calling in reference to …"
      ii. "Hi _____. This is _____, how is everything going?"
      iii. "Hi _____, it's _____. Wondered if you'd like to see a movie?"
   b. Closing
      i. "It was great talking with you – talk to you again soon."
      ii. "Thanks for your help. Goodbye."
      iii. "Oh, I hear my doorbell – I'd better go now."

Preparing to Answer a Call

1. Arrange for Caller ID, if possible, so you will know in advance who is calling. If you have an answering machine, you have the option of answering the call when the phone rings or letting the person calling leave a message and then calling back when you are ready.
2. Have pen and pad available by the phone at all times.
3. Have some opening responses available:
   a. "Oh, _____. It's good to hear from you."
   b. "Hello, _____. I'm glad you called."
   c. "Thank you for returning my call."

> **Tip:** Cue cards are helpful.

Keeping Track of Phone Messages

Use an organized message pad such as the one below to ensure that you get the information you need in a format that is easy to refer to at a later date.

Day and date	Name & phone number of caller	Message	Response	Follow-up needed

From E. S. Korin (2007). *Asperger Syndrome – An Owner's Manual 2.* Shawnee Mission, KS: Autism Asperger Publishing Company; www.asperger.net. Used with permission.

Travel

Preparing to travel is exciting but can also be stressful. Being organized (preparing and planning) can alleviate some of the anxiety and help promote positive anticipatory feelings.
You can find checklists to help you prepare on line at sites such as www.GoFox.com (click on Travel Tools at the bottom of the page) or www.cruisecritic.com or do a search for "travel checklists."

Doctor's Appointments

One of the life skills older adolescents and adults must develop is the ability to maintain their health and to manage their health issues. This is a brief, but helpful list of how to set up and conduct a doctor's appointment. Additional lists you might consult include ordering and managing medications, what to expect during hospitalization or trips to the emergency room.

Call to schedule appointment
- Write the appointment in a calendar or planner
- Get directions if needed
- Before you go, write down:
    - Questions you want to ask
    - Medications you are taking
    - Concerns you want to talk about

Bring
- Directions
- List of questions
- List of concerns
- Your insurance card
- Money for co-pay and parking (if appropriate)

Before you leave
- Make next appointment
- Get prescriptions
- Get referrals if needed

Bill Paying

As discussed in the section on controlling clutter and organizing (page 64), go through your mail daily to maintain order and prevent becoming overwhelmed. On each bill that arrives, write the due date on the front of the envelope and file it in a mail holder in a prominent location on the top of your work space (desk) or put it in a specially designed folder. Overdue bills are expensive, and consistently late payment can harm your credit rating.

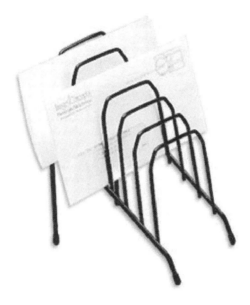

- Pick a regular time each week to review bills. Put this on your weekly calendar and stick to this routine.

- Go through your bills and pay them.

- Make sure to have stamps.

- Put bills in a visible location (near door, near keys) in order to remember to mail them (or pay online).

- Submit for payment.

Independent Life Skills Assessments

Comprehensive assessments of readiness for adult life may be found at www.dshs.wa.gov (Washington State Department of Social and Health Services) and http://www.caseylifeskills.org/

Here you will find free and easy-to-use tools to help young people prepare for adulthood. The life skills assessments provide instant feedback.

Career Planning

http://www.myfuture.com/
This is an excellent source of information for planning your future.

My Future is a service presented by the United States Department of Defense (DoD).

Its stated goal is to help students understand the opportunities available to them after graduation and better prepare them for the choices and challenges they have ahead.

Although it is theoretically promoting the military as a career option, the site has lots of good information.

Resources Related to Asperger Syndrome and Autism Spectrum Disorders in General

Excellent booklists and other information related to autism spectrum disorders and Asperger Syndrome are located at the following websites:

    www.amazon.com keywords: autism, autism spectrum disorders, Asperger Syndrome
    www.asperger.net
    www.aane.org

Additional information may be obtained at the following websites.

ASPERGER HELP

http://aspergerhelp.net
The mission of Asperger Help is to be a center for people seeking answers, sharing knowledge, understanding the process, and educating others about several disorders on the spectrum such as Autism, Aspergers, ADHD, Tourettes, and more.

YALE DEVELOPMENTAL DISABILITIES CLINIC

http://info.med.yale.edu/chldstudy/autism/index.html
The Yale Developmental Disabilities Clinic offers comprehensive, multidisciplinary evaluations for children with social disabilities, usually focusing on the issues of diagnosis and intervention. The clinic is headed by Fred Volkmar, M.D., and Ami Klin, Ph.D., two of the most respected experts in the field of autism, Asperger's Syndrome (AS), and other Pervasive Developmental Disorders (PDDs). We are also conducting several large research projects on autism, AS, and other PDDs. The clinic is located in the Child Study Center at Yale University in New Haven, Connecticut.

AANE

www.aane.com
Asperger Association of New England
Great resource for information, resources and contacts. Great site for anyone interested in ASD – not just people in New England.

ASPEN

www.aspennj.org
ASPEN® provides families and individuals whose lives are affected by autism spectrum disorders (Asperger Syndrome, pervasive developmental disorder-NOS, high-functioning autism), and nonverbal learning disabilities with:

- Education about the issues surrounding the disorders.
- Support in knowing that they are not alone, and in helping individuals with ASDs and NLD achieve their maximum potential.
- Advocacy in areas of appropriate educational programs, medical research funding, adult issues and increased public awareness and understanding.

THE SOURCE

www.asperger.org

MAAP Services for Autism and Asperger Syndrome is a nonprofit organization dedicated to providing information and advice to families of More advanced individuals with Autism, Asperger syndrome, and Pervasive developmental disorder (PDD).

AUTISM SOCIETY OF AMERICA

www.autism-society.org

The Autism Society of America (ASA) is dedicated to increasing public awareness about autism and the day-to-day issues faced by individuals with autism, their families and the professionals with whom they interact. ASA and its local chapters share a common mission of providing information and education, supporting research and advocating for programs and services for the autism community.

CENTER FOR THE STUDY FOR AUTISM

www.autism.org

www.autism-resources.com

A collaborative of several organizations involved in the study of autism.

THE NATIONAL AUTISTIC SOCIETY (UK)

www.nas.org.uk

The National Autistic Society (NAS) champions the rights and interests of all people with autism and ensures that they and their families receive quality services appropriate to their needs. The website includes information about autism and Asperger Syndrome, as well as NAS and its services and activities.

NATIONAL INSTITUTES OF HEALTH

www.nimh.nih.gov

Click on "Health Information"

Click on "Autism Spectrum Disorders (Pervasive Developmental Disorders)"

The National Institutes of Health (NIH), a part of the U.S. Department of Health and Human Services, is the primary federal agency for conducting and supporting medical research. Helping to lead the way toward important medical discoveries that improve people's health and save lives, NIH scientists investigate ways to prevent disease as well as the causes, treatments, and even cures for common and rare diseases.

NLD (Nonverbal Learning Disorder) ON THE WEB

www.nldontheweb.org

A comprehensive source of information on nonverbal learning disabilities for parents and professionals. Includes full-text articles and other important resources.

THE SHYNESS INSTITUTE

www.shyness.com

Gathering of network resources for people seeking information and services for shyness.

WRONG PLANET

www.wrongplanet.net

A meeting place for people on the spectrum or thereabouts.

Other books from
Autism Asperger Publishing Company
focusing on adolescents and adults

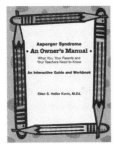

Asperger Syndrome – An Owner's Manual: What You, Your Parents and Your Teachers Need to Know; An Interactive Guide and Workbook

Ellen S. Heller Korin

Code 9960 **Price: $17.95**

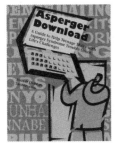

Asperger Download: A Guide for Teenage Males with Asperger Syndrome

Josie and Damian Santomauro

Code 9990 **Price: $19.95**

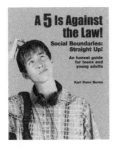

A 5 Is Against the Law! Social Boundaries: Straight Up! An honest guide for teens and young adults

Kari Dunn Buron

Code 9975 **Price: $19.95**

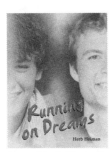

Running on Dreams

Herb Heiman

Code 9972 (fiction) **Price: $18.95**

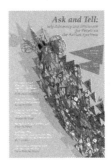

Ask and Tell: Self-Advocacy and Disclosure for People on the Autism Spectrum

Edited by Stephen M. Shore; foreword by Temple Grandin; contributing authors: Ruth Elaine Hane, Kassiane Sibley, Stephen M. Shore, Roger N. Meyer, Phil Schwarz, Liane Holliday Willey

Code 9940 **Price: $21.95**

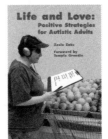

Life and Love: Positive Strategies for Autistic Adults

Zosia Zaks

Code 9965 **Price $24.95**

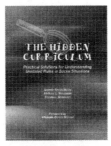

The Hidden Curriculum: Practical Solutions for Understanding Unstated Rules in Social Situations

Brenda Smith Myles, Melissa L. Trautman, and Ronda L. Schelvan

Code 9942 (book) **Price: $19.95**
Code 9721 (DVD) **Price: $29.95**
One-A-Day Calendar **Price: $15.95**

To order:
Autism Asperger Publishing Co.
P.O. Box 23173
Shawnee Mission, Kansas 66283-0173
877-277-8254
www.asperger.net

APC

Autism Asperger Publishing Co.
P.O. Box 23173
Shawnee Mission, Kansas 66283-0173
www.asperger.net